M.C.Q. TUT OR FOR
ANAESTH

M.C.Q. TUTOR FOR ANAESTHETISTS

A. W. GROGONO, MD, FFARCS
Associate Professor, Department of Anaesthesiology, State University of New York, Upstate Medical Center, Syracuse.
Formerly Consultant Anaesthetist,
Royal Free Hospital, London

and

T. HILARY HOWELLS, MB, BS, FFARCS
Director, Department of Anaesthesia, Royal Free Hospital, London

WILLIAM HEINEMANN MEDICAL BOOKS LIMITED
London

First published 1975

Reprinted 1977

© A. W. Grogono and T. H. Howells 1975

ISBN 0 433 12625 6

Text set in 10/11 pt IBM Century, printed by photolithography,
and bound in Great Britain at The Pitman Press, Bath

CONTENTS

PREFACE

This book is called a Tutor because its primary aim is to be an aid to teaching and learning. The value of the multiple choice question (M.C.Q.) in this educational role has been convincingly demonstrated in our departmental primary F.F.A.R.C.S. tutorials and in our six-monthly Final F.F.A. course. The discussion provoked by each question and by consideration of the possible answers allowed the relevant subject to be thoroughly discussed. This led to improvements and modifications to our original bank of questions as well as generating new ideas which allowed the bank to be enlarged. The discussion notes which accompany every question also stem from these tutorials, confirmed and amplified where necessary by reference to standard text books.

During the time that we have been using M.C.Q.s in teaching and for in-course assessment, they have been introduced into the Primary F.F.A.R.C.S. examination. Although they have proved their value here*, there are as yet no plans to incorporate a similar section into the Final part. With the Primary candidate in mind, answer sheets have been prepared which allow a reader to practise answering questions.

It is a pleasure to record the help we have received from Dr. Janet Hoare, Dr. Nicholas Norwell and Dr. Margaret Robertson who have scrutinized, investigated, modified and written many of the questions and answers, to thank our secretary Miss Ann Toogood for her endless patience and to thank Mr. Owen Evans of Heinemann's for his help and encouragement.

A.W.G.
T.H.H.

*Hunter, A. R. (1974). *Proc. Roy. Soc. Med.*, 67, 173.

INTRODUCTION

Multiple choice questions are increasingly being used in the assessment and examination of candidates in a wide variety of subjects. Until recently, medical examinations have usually been based on a mixture of written essays, clinical examinations and vivas. Despite the attractions, and possibly even the relevance, of such examination methods, they all suffer from the disadvantage that they provide no reproduceable results. An examiner remarking papers after an interval is unable even to reproduce a previous assessment of pass or fail, far less rank them reliably in descending order of merit. In contrast, a set of multiple choice questions drawn from a relevant and adequately prepared collection will rank the candidates fairly consistently. The precision with which the examination achieves this discrimination is improved by using only "ideal" questions at the "pass" level of difficulty but the penalty incurred is that there will be less reliable ranking because (theoretically at least) all the candidates who pass should obtain 100 per cent. In practice there is no such group of ideal questions and candidates find some questions easy, some difficult and some impossible.

A candidate often feels resentment against M.C.Q.s because they allow no room for explanation and demand an unequivocal answer. In addition he may feel that in medicine it is often as important to know what should be avoided, or what must not be done, as it is to know the "correct" answer. Until recently the format of many answer sheets precluded the candidate from displaying such negative knowledge and this source of irritation was not entirely removed by reassurance that "statistically it made little difference" which way each question, and thus his knowledge, was scored. Answer marking which allows the candidate to display his knowledge of both correct and incorrect alternatives are therefore to be preferred; such answer sheets have been included in this book for use with the questions.

Examiners may also feel resentment against M.C.Q.s because they find them such hard taskmasters to produce. Sensible distractors are hard to invent; qualifying words like "mostly" or "usually" must be avoided, and ambiguity and errors must be sought and eliminated. After the paper has been marked the examination analysis identifies some questions as too easy, some as

vii

too hard and others as apparently irrelevant to the particular set of questions in use, and there is consequently an unending requirement for extra questions.

However, despite reservations of candidate and examiner, M.C.Q.s will undoubtedly be used for many years to come and candidates should approach such an exam with knowledge of the technique and preferably with some practical experience.

The five-alternative question used in this book is representative of those suitable for testing factual knowledge in a scientific subject. Various other multiple choice question formats have been employed with the intention of additionally testing logic or reasoning ability. These do not form an important part of most medical examinations but when employed there is usually a group of such questions preceded by a clear explanation of how to answer them. Some questions in this book consist of five independent statements preceded by "Which of the following are true:" but most questions consist of a "stem", or incomplete statement/ question, with five alternatives following it. In some examinations the candidate is told that there will always be only one correct answer. The candidate finds this attractive as it makes guessing easier, tending to forget that his neighbour benefits too. For our questions any number of alternatives may be correct, including on some occasions no correct answers and on others all five answers correct. Some questions of course clearly invite only one answer: "Atmospheric pressure expressed in cm H_2O is approximately" implies that only one alternative is correct.

In addition to their established position in assessment and examination, multiple choice questions can make a further contribution to the education process. Whatever the subject there is no one method of learning, revising and keeping up to date which suits everybody, and even for any one individual it is probably inefficient to use one method of learning exclusively; the additional stimulus which variety provides is particularly useful when an element of challenge or test is included. Thus, however good a text book is, it is unlikely to be used to its best advantage unless the reader is also stimulated by questions, challenged by tutorials or tested in vivas. Many an anaesthetist in training is well supplied with such additional stimuli. Departmental meetings, instruction in the operating theatre, discussion with colleagues and intermittent exposure to examinations may provide sufficient incentive to make him read the text books. Not everyone is so fortunate. Some anaesthetists, whether trained or in training, experience too little challenge to stimulate them to further reading. In this situation it is hard to reach the standard required by an examination and even harder to maintain that standard when examinations are completed.

A set of multiple choice questions is a useful adjunct to learning, and one which is adaptable to the needs of the individual. The beginner can work slowly and use the questions to stimulate him to read; the advanced student can test his ability to answer questions at speed under exam conditions; the teacher can quickly review a wide range of subjects choosing some for discussion and others for revision.

In the following pages every question is supported not only by the answer but also by a short discussion or explanation. This allows the inclusion of some additional material, and it provides an opportunity to comment on the incorrect answers as well as on the correct. A well-prepared candidate may know the subject and will then be able to reassure himself from the answer and the explanation and move quickly to the next question. His less well-informed colleague may find that the explanation is no more sufficient than was merely discovering the correct answer. It is for this reason that we recommend that this book is used in conjunction with standard texts.

Readers are advised to detach and complete the answer sheets which they will find at the back of the book. This self-discipline to make a decision is useful practice for examinations, helps the reader to concentrate and provides a convenient check list when turning the page to consider the answers.

Questions have been divided into main subjects, although this has necessitated some arbitrary allocation. Each question is printed on the right-hand side of the page with the correct answers and commentary on the following page. The commentary on each question is necessarily brief; the well-informed reader should find his memory adequately refreshed while others should seek further information from other sources.

In contrast to the time which may be devoted to the questions and answers in this book where the main objective has been education, when sitting a multiple choice question test candidates should avoid devoting too much time to early questions. No marks are awarded for unanswered questions at the end, and amongst these questions there may be easy questions completed in a few seconds. In addition, selections should not be recorded on the basis of guesswork as this usually affects the score adversely. Readers should bear these points in mind if they wish to score the answer sheets provided.

1. ANATOMY

1.1. Features of the stellate ganglion block include:

   A. Exophthalmos
   B. Lack of sweating in the ipselateral face and neck
   C. Miosis
   D. Ptosis
   E. Congestion in the contralateral nares.

1.2. When an axillary brachial plexus block is performed:

   A. 10 ml of 1% lignocaine is adequate
   B. The deltoid muscle may be penetrated
   C. Cutaneous sensation is not abolished over the medial
      side of the arm
   D. Pneumothorax is a complication
   E. The point of injection is between the insertions of pec-
      toralis major and latissimus dorsi.

1.3. The inferior dental nerve:

   A. Is the largest branch of the mandibular nerve
   B. Gives off the nerve to mylohyoid
   C. Carries motor supply to orbicularis oris
   D. Carries secreto-motor fibres to sub-mandibular salivary
      gland
   E. Carries sensory fibres from the anterior two-thirds of
      the tongue.

Answers overleaf

1

1.1. B, C, D.

All signs are, of course, on the side of the block. Horner's syndrome triad is enophthalmos, ptosis and miosis. Nasal congestion (Guttmann's sign) and anhidrosis are frequent accompaniments. The occurrence of Horner's syndrome does not guarantee successful sympathetic block in the arm.

1.2. C, E.

At least 20—25 ml of 1% lignocaine is needed to fill the axillary sheath even when spread is limited by tourniquet. No brachial block will ablate sensation in the media area of the upper arm which is supplied by T.2. Neither pneumothorax nor phrenic block complicate the axillary approach to the plexus.

1.3. A, B.

After giving a branch to the mylohyoid muscle, the inferior dental continues as wholly somatic sensory. General sensation to the anterior two-thirds of the tongue is supplied by the lingual nerve which also carries fibres from chorda tympani that are secreto-motor to sub-mandibular and sub-lingual salivary glands, and which carry taste from the anterior two-thirds of the tongue.

Anatomy

1.4. The innervation of the human larynx is such that:

   A. The internal laryngeal branch of the superior laryngeal branch of the vagus supplies the lingual surface of the epiglottis

   B. In the cadaveric position the cords are fully abducted

   C. Total bilateral recurrent nerve palsy leads to severe adductor spasm

   D. The glossopharyngeal nerves are sensory to the laryngeal mucous membrane above the level of the vocal cords

   E. The recurrent laryngeal nerves are sensory to the laryngeal mucous membrane below the level of the vocal cords.

1.5. Which of the following nerves supply the intrinsic muscles of the larynx:

   A. Internal laryngeal

   B. Hypoglossal

   C. Those originating in the nucleus ambiguous

   D. Recurrent laryngeal

   E. Glossopharyngeal.

1.6. The segmental innervation of the human genital tract involves:

   A. Motor nerves to the body of the uterus from T.5—10

   B. Motor nerves to the cervix from L.2, 3, 4

   C. Sensory nerves from the body of the uterus to T.11 and T.12

   D. Sensory nerves from the cervix to S.2, 3, 4

   E. Sensory nerves from the vagina to L.5, S.1.

1.7. The knee jerk:

   A. Is mediated through spinal segments L.2, 3, 4

   B. Is mediated through receptors in the patellar tendon

   C. Is mediated through receptors in the quadriceps muscle

   D. Is a monosynaptic reflex

   E. Is diminished in upper motor neurone lesion.

Answers overleaf

1.4. E.

The lingual surface of the epiglottis is supplied by the glossopharyngeal nerve. The cords cannot fully abduct without activity in such muscles as the cricothyroid. Bilateral recurrent laryngeal nerve damage leads to severe spasm because abductor fibres are more vulnerable than adductors, allowing adductor dominance. When the nerves are severed totally, although adduction predominates, the cords do not seriously obstruct ventilation unless inspiratory effort is increased. Laryngeal sensation is supplied by internal and recurrent laryngeal nerves, above and below cords respectively.

1.5. C, D.

All the intrinsic muscles of the larynx are supplied by the recurrent laryngeal nerves with the exception of the crico-thyroid which is supplied by the external laryngeal branch of the superior laryngeal nerve (which also serves the inferior pharyngeal constrictor). The nucleus ambiguous is the viscero-motor centre in the floor of the 4th ventricle. The internal laryngeal nerve is sensory to the mucous membrane above the vocal cords. The hypoglossal is the motor nerve of the tongue and the glossopharyngeal supplies motor and sensory fibres above the level of the larynx.

1.6. A, C, D.

Thus, sensory block up to T.10 is ideal for labour pain relief without effecting a motor paralysis. Nevertheless, block up to T.6 as for Caesarean section does not appear to impede uterine contractions. S.2, 3, 4 serve the lower birth canal (pudendal nerve) and lower uterine segment and cervix.

1.7. A, C, D.

Stretch receptors acually lie in the quadriceps muscle. No connector cell is involved between the sensory and motor neurones. Upper motor neurone lesions characteristically exaggerate tendon reflexes.

1.8. Parasympathetic outflow is carried by:

    A. The IIIrd cranial nerve
    B. The VIIth cranial nerve
    C. The glossopharyngeal nerve
    D. The facial nerve
    E. The 2nd and 3rd sacral nerves.

1.9. Which of the following structures receive pre-ganglionic sympathetic fibres:

    A. The coelic ganglion
    B. The adrenal medulla
    C. The otic ganglion
    D. The nervi erigentes
    E. The carotid body.

1.10. The diaphragm:

    A. Has origins from the lower six ribs
    B. Is pierced at T.12 level by the oesophagus
    C. Is pierced at T.10 level by the aorta
    D. Receives sensory nerve supply from the lower six intercostal nerves
    E. May refer pain to the shoulder if periphery is involved.

1.11. Concerning the brachial plexus:

    A. Its roots lie deep to the anterior scalene
    B. Its cords lie in the posterior triangle of the neck
    C. It gives origin to the musculo-cutaneous nerve of the arm
    D. Its posterior cord continues as the radial nerve
    E. The suprascapular nerves arise from the trunks.

Answers overleaf

1. 8. A, B, C, D, E.

The facial nerve is the VIIth cranial! The vagus is the only other cranial parasympathetic carrier. The sacral nerves mentioned complete the entire parasympathetic outflow from the C.N.S.

1.9. A, B.

The coeliac ganglion and adrenal medulla both receive preganglionic sympathetic fibres. The otic ganglion is a parasympathetic relay centre but receives postganglionic sympathetic transits. The nervi erigentes comprise the sacral parasympathetic outflow. The carotid body receives both types of autonomic post-ganglionic fibres and is densely innervated.

1.10. A, D.

The diaphragm is pierced by the oesophagus at T.10 and by the aorta at T.12. The lower six intercostal nerves carry sensation from the periphery and account for "stitch" pain. The phrenic nerves carry sensation from the central diaphragm and may refer pain to the shoulder.

1.11. A, C, D, E.

The cords lie around the axillary artery, the trunks in the posterior triangle of the neck. The musculo-cutaneous nerve is given off the lateral cord. (The plexus supplies the entire arm with the exception of a skin area over the medial upper arm which receives sensory supply from the intercosto-brachial nerve from T.2.)

1.12. The pudendal nerve:

    A. Arises from L.2, 3, 4
    B. Crosses the greater sciatic foramen
    C. Crosses the lesser sciatic foramen
    D. Gives off the inferior haemorrhoidal nerve
    E. Gives off the dorsal nerve of the penis.

Answers overleaf

1.12. B, C, D, E.

This nerve arises from S.2, 3, 4. It crosses both sciatic foramina and is conveniently blocked in its canal, a fascial tunnel on the outer wall of the ischio-rectal fossa.

2. ANAESTHESIA AND EQUIPMENT

2.1. Untoward reflex effects of surgical traction on the extrinsic muscles of the eye (e.g. during correction of strabismus) are satisfactorily avoided using:

  A. Suxamethonium
  B. Gallamine
  C. Tubocurarine
  D. Hyoscine
  E. Facial nerve block.

2.2. 200 ml per minute of oxygen are passed through a copper kettle vaporizer containing halothane. When the total gas flow from the anaesthetic machine is 5 litres per minute, then the expected halothane vapour concentration will be approximately:

  A. 2.0%
  B. 1.33%
  C. 0.67%
  D. 0.5%
  E. 0.33%

2.3. Curarization may be prolonged by the presence of:

  A. Streptomycin
  B. Neomycin
  C. Polymyxin
  D. Tetracycline
  E. Kanamycin.

Answers overleaf

2.1. B.

Question refers to bradycardia, cardiac arrest and arrhythmias due to oculocardiac reflex. Gallamine is useful because of its vagolytic cardiac action. This complication may also be avoided using atropine intravenously or by retro-orbital injection of local anaesthetic.

2.2. A.

The saturated vapour concentration of halothane at room temperature is 241 mmHg (about $\frac{1}{3}$ atmosphere). As a kettle delivers saturated vapour, halothane wil be $\frac{1}{3}$ of the volume and the fresh gas will occupy the remaining volume $\frac{2}{3}$. Thus the 200 ml fresh gas must be joined by 100 ml halothane. This is 1/50 (2%) of the total flow.

2.3. A, B, C, E.

Neuromuscular block can be caused by streptomycin, neomycin, polymyxin, kanamycin and dihydrostreptomycin, and possibly by rolitetracycline and by bacitracin. This block is competitive and is enhanced by the presence of tubocurarine and other competitive nueromuscular blockers. Tetracycline and penicillin are not implicated. The other antobiotics mentioned exert their neuromuscular effect by reducing calcium ions at the end-plate.

2.4. There are contraindications to the use of suxamethonium in patients with:

A. Epilepsy
B. Pyrexia
C. Hyperkalaemia
D. Hypokalaemia
E. Severe burns

2.5. The intensity of the neuromuscular block produced by tubo-curarine and gallamine is influenced by hyperventilation as follows:

A. Intensity of both increased
B. Tubocurarine increased, gallamine decreased
C. Tubocurarine decreased, gallamine increased
D. Intensity of both decreased
E. No effect on intensity of either.

2.6. In well-managed induced hypothermia to 30°C:

A. There is a decrease in blood viscosity
B. The CO_2 content of arterial blood tends to rise
C. There is resistance to suxamethonium
D. Hyperglycaemia may exist
E. The circulation may be safely arrested for seven minutes.

2.7. Pulmonary oedema may result from the following impurities in a nitrous oxide cylinder:

A. Nitrogen
B. Nitric oxide
C. Nitrogen dioxide
D. Steel dust in the cylinder
E. Carbon monoxide.

Answers overleaf

2.4. C, E.

Massive depolarization with release of intracellular potassium may be dangerous in hyperkalaemic patients (such as those with severe burns).

2.5. C.

In healthy volunteers hyperventilation reduces the effect of tubocurarine and enhances that of gallamine. Hypoventilation causes the reverse. This provides a rational basis for preferring gallamine when small doses are given during spontaneous ventilation ("A touch of Flax") and for choosing tubocurarine during hyperventilation. In both cases the neuromuscular block decreases reliably as time passes.

2.6. B, D, E.

There may be hyperglycaemia due to diminished insulin release and diminished liver metabolism. The CO_2 content is high because low temperature increases solubility and buffer activity. Blood viscosity increases. There is sensitivity to suxamethonium. The circulation may be arrested for seven minutes.

2.7. B, C.

Nitrous oxide is manufactured by heating ammonium nitrate:

$$NH_4NO_3 \rightarrow N_2O + 2H_2O.$$

The impurities which may arise are: NO_2, N_2O_3, N_2, NH_3, HNO_3, H_2O. It is the higher oxides of nitrogen which may cause pulmonary oedema. Impurities are normally removed by passing the gas through water, acid, potassium permanganate and a liquifier.

2.8. The size of a cubicle for intensive therapy should be at least:

    A. 80 sq ft
    B. 200 sq ft
    C. 500 sq ft
    D. 600 cu ft
    E. 800 cu ft.

2.9. It would be correct for the following pieces of endobronchial equipment to have a cuff inflated in the left main bronchus:

    A. The Vernon Thompson endobronchial blocker
    B. The Green-Gordon tube
    C. The Macintosh-Leatherdale tube
    D. The Carlens tube
    E. The Vellacott tube.

2.10. A suitable local analgesic for infiltration of the skin of the abdomen for an abdominal incision would be:

    A. 0.1% lignocaine with 1:200,000 adrenaline
    B. 1.0% lignocaine with 1:100,000 adrenaline
    C. 0.5% lignocaine with 1:200,000 adrenaline
    D. 0.5% lignocaine
    E. 0.5% bupivicaine.

Answers overleaf

2.8. B.

The recommended size is between 180 and 400 sq ft. In a room 250 to 300 sq ft, with the bed against the wall this is equivalent to an 8 ft space between the bed and the other walls, a space frequently required by equipment (ventilators, mobile X-ray equipment, monitoring equipment, nursing trolleys), for minor surgery (tracheostomy), for resuscitation and for transferring patients to and from stretchers and other beds.

2.9. A, C, D.

The high position of the right upper lobe bronchus leaves insufficient space for a simple cuff to provide an airtight junction between a tube and the whole right lung. Accordingly, the single lumen Macintosh-Leatherdale and the double lumen Carlens tube were all designed with a cuff to be inflated in the (longer) left main bronchus. The single lumen right-sided tubes Vellacott and Green-Gordon both have cuffs inflated at the level of the right upper lobe bronchus; the Green-Gordon cuff incorporates an orifice to the right upper lobe and is thus used to ventilate the entire right lung. The Vellacott cuff seals the right upper lobe but appropriate orifices permit ventilation of the remainder of both lungs. Thompson and Magill blockers may be used for any bronchus wide enough to accept them.

2.10. C, D.

The volume required necessitates a low anaesthetic concentration to minimise the risk of toxicity and a low adrenaline concentration to minimise cardiac effects.

2.11. The use of muscle relaxants is affected when anaesthetizing:

A. Neonates
B. Patients receiving frusemide
C. Patients with porphyria
D. Patients under hypothermia
E. Patients with penetrating injuries of the eye.

Answers overleaf

2.11. A, B, D, E.

Neonates are sensitive to tubocurarine and other competitive blockers. Frusemide depletes body potassium and if not replaced, the resulting hypokalaemia will enhance the action of non-depolarizing agents. Although porphyria may be associated with low plasma sodium and potassium, the use of muscle relaxants is not affected. As patients are cooled, large doses of tubocurarine are required to maintain effective neuromuscular block. This is not metabolized, and during rewarming profound curarization may be encountered. Intra-ocular contents may be expelled through the wound by the suxamethonium contraction.

2.12. When there is a reduction in the fresh gas flow supplying a Magill (Mapleson "A") circuit used for spontaneous ventilation, there will be an inverse relationship between the fresh gas flow and the rise in the patient's PCO_2 if the fresh gas flow falls below:

A. Twice the patient's minute volume
B. Twice the patient's alveolar ventilation
C. The patient's minute volume
D. The patient's alveolar ventilation
E. Two-thirds of the patient's alveolar ventilation.

Answers overleaf

2.12. D.

To avoid CO_2 retention *at least* the alveolar ventilation must be displaced from the circuit every minute. Without CO_2 absorption therefore the fresh gas flow should be more than the alveolar ventilation. At lower fresh gas flows the rise in CO_2 is inversely proportional to the fresh gas flow. The behaviour of this circuit can be understood best by considering an example.

The diagram represents the Magill circuit in use in a patient breathing 20 times a minute (1 second inspiration, 1 second expiration, 1 second pause) at a tidal volume of 450 ml (minute volume 9 litres) supplied with a fresh gas flow equal to his alveolar ventilation (6 litres per minute). The patient has completed exhalation (end of 2nd second).

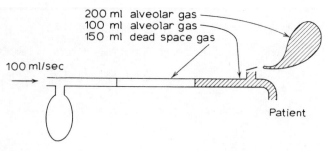

By the end of the 2nd second 200 ml of fresh gas will have entered the circuit. Thus, of the 450 ml he exhales, 200 ml will have to leave via the pressure relief valve. 150 ml of dead space (unused) gas will have entered the hose first, followed by 100 ml of alveolar gas. During the pause, this latter gas will be driven out by the fresh gas flow.

In clinical practice it is wise to exceed slightly the theoretical minimum of making the fresh gas flow equal to the alveolar ventilation; this allows for errors in minute volume estimation as well as for some mixing of gases. Excessive fresh gas flows result in wastage and unnecessary pollution.

2.13. The soda lime used to absorb CO_2 in anaesthesia:

    A. Generates water during the reaction
    B. Requires water for the reaction to occur
    C. Absorbs heat during the reaction
    D. Is composed mainly of sodium hydroxide
    E. Has its hardness improved by the addition of potassium hydroxide.

For each of the questions 2.14 — 2.18 select the best answer only:

    2.14. Tends to maintain the tidal volume despite the appearance of a leak in the circuit
    2.15. Tends to maintain tidal volume despite changes in compliance
    2.16. Tends to produce "square topped" ("plateau") type of pressure wave
    2.17. Cannot be time-cycled
    2.18. Tends to maintain inspiratory flow rate despite changes in airway resistance.

    A. Flow generators
    B. Pressure generators
    C. Volume pre-set
    D. Pressure pre-set
    E. None of the above.

Answers overleaf

2.13. A, B.

Although water is generated by the reaction:

$$Ca(OH)_2 + CO_2 \rightarrow CaCO_3 + H_2O,$$

the reaction requires the presence of some water. Heat is produced. The composition is approximately 5% NaOH, 90% $Ca(OH)_2$. KOH is added to improve absorption. Hardness is improved by the addition of silicates. In addition to these (dry) components there is about 14—19% water.

2.14-D; 2.15-C; 2.11-B; 2.17-E; 2.18-A.

These classifications make it possible to anitcipate a ventilator's response to changes in the patient (compliance and airway resistance), i.e. "Will the breathing be affected?" *N.B.* Each classification applies to only one aspect of breathing:

Classification	*Only applies to:*
Flow versus *Pressure* generator	Inspiratory flow
Volume versus *Pressure* pre-set	Tidal volume
Minute volume pre-set or not	Minute volume.

In effect, each classification supplies equivalent information; the ventilator is either able to resist a change in the patient ("stable") or it yields ("flexible"). Each classification is *independent* of the others. None by itself precludes time-cycling, although a pair may, e.g. a pressure pre-set flow generator cannot additionally be time-cycled. Question 2.14 concerns tidal volume; only the volume pre-set/pressure pre-set distinction is applicable; a leak should normally be corrected but when present the tidal volume is more likely to be maintained by a ventilator which continues to produce its pre-set pressure.

2.19. When a patient is breathing from a closed circuit (circle) the vaporizer may be in the circle (V.I.C.) or outside in the fresh gas supply line (V.O.C.). Which of the following situations will cause the inspired vapour concentration to rise:

    A. V.I.C., decreased minute volume
    B. V.I.C., decreased fresh gas flow
    C. V.O.C., increased minute volume
    D. V.O.C., increased fresh gas flow
    E. None of the above.

2.20. During hypothermia:

    A. Curare is potentiated
    B. Action of suxamethonium is reduced
    C. For a given PCO_2 level, the pH tends to be lower
    D. Haemoglobin releases oxygen to the tissues less easily
    E. Intravenous glucose should be given.

2.21. The first direct-vision laryngoscope was devised by:

    A. Magill
    B. Guedel
    C. Macintosh
    D. Kirstein
    E. Hewitt.

Answers overleaf

2.19. B, D.

When a vaporizer is *in* the closed circuit (V.I.C.), an increase in the minute volume causes the gas in the closed circuit to pass more frequently through the vaporizer and the vapour concentration in the circuit rises. Fresh gas dilutes the vapour concentration so that a fall in the fresh gas flow allows the concentration to rise. The reverse is true when the supply of vapour depends on the fresh gas flow (V.O.C.). The effect on the concentration can be represented:

	Fresh gas ↑	Min. Vol. ↑
V.I.C	↓	↑
V.O.C.	↑	↓

2.20. C, D.

Hypothermia reduces the block due to curare. Any increased dosage may cause prolonged curarization on rewarming. The magnitude and duration of the block due to suxamethonium is increased. Increased solubility means that for a given PCO_2 more carbon dioxide is dissolved with an associated rise in the hydrogen ion concentration (low pH). This acidity would normally shift the oxygen dissociation curve to the right (to help unload oxygen) but hypothermia overrides this effect and the curve moves to the left so that haemoglobin unloads its oxygen *less* readily. The hypothermic liver metabolises glucose slowly and intravenous glucose should be avoided.

2.21. D.

Kirstein devised the first direct-vision laryngoscope in 1895. Magill described his straight blade laryngoscope in 1926 and Macintosh his curved blade in 1943. Guedel published on signs of anaesthesia in 1920 and described his airway in 1933. Hewitt invented the first practical gas and air machine in 1887 and described his airway in 1908.

2.22. Trichlorethylene vaporizers for use by midwives should not supply more of the agent than:

A. 0.07%
B. 0.1%
C. 0.2%
D. 0.5%
E. 0.7%

2.23. Halothane in clinical concentration:

A. Is flammable
B. Causes enzyme induction
C. Is all excreted unchanged
D. Does not stimulate the production of endogenous catecholamines
E. Is not absorbed by rubber.

2.24. In Britain anaesthesia was first administered for a surgical operation in:

A. 1824
B. 1842
C. 1846
D. 1864
E. 1884.

2.25. A slow pulse during halothane anaesthesia may be due to:

A. A-V nodal rhythm
B. Vagal action at S-A node
C. Idio-ventricular rhythm
D. Multiple ventricular extrasystoles
E. Bigeminal rhythm.

Answers overleaf

23

2.22. D.

Midwives are permitted to administer up to 0.5% trichlorethylene. Vaporizers should be temperature compensated as temperature variation affects the vapour pressure and hence the concentration. The Emotril and Tecota Mk 6 satisfy the requirements.

2.23. B, D.

Halothane is only flammable in hyperbaric oxygen/nitrous oxide mixtures. It causes induction of hepatic microsomal enzymes and is itself metabolized. Its metabolism is enhanced in patients on barbiturates and other enzyme inducers. It does not stimulate catecholamine production, although associated carbon dioxide retention may do so. It is highly soluble in rubber.

2.24. C.

1824 Animals operated on by Hickman using CO_2.
1842 Ether administered in America.
1846 Squire administered ether to Frederick Churchill for amputation by Liston in U.C.H.
1864 Chloroform committee reported favourably.
1884 Cocaine's use for surface anaesthesia of the cornea demonstrated by Köller, and for conduction anaesthesia of the mandibular nerve demonstrated by Halstead and Hall.

2.25. A, B, C, D, E.

Any of these may cause bradycardia, although bigeminal rhythm is more characteristic of digitalis overdose. The commonest arrhythmias with halothane are A-V nodal rhythm and ventricular extrasystoles.

2.26. Air embolism:

    A. May be treated by placing the patient on the right side
    B. Is more dangerous in the presence of a ventricular septal defect
    C. Can be detected using ultrasound
    D. Commonly causes initial hyperventilation
    E. May be treated by hyperbaric oxygen therapy.

Answers overleaf

2.26. B, C, D, E.

Air embolism blocks blood flow in capillary beds (e.g. in the lung). Small bubbles of air can be detected by their ability to reflect ultrasound.

Air in the right side of the heart interferes with normal pumping and can be detected by auscultation (the mill wheel murmur).

Hyperbaric treatment compresses the bubbles and oxygen therapy (no inspired nitrogen) allows reduction of blood nitrogen tension and therefore also aids reabsorption of bubbles.

3. CLINICAL PATHOLOGY AND BIOCHEMISTRY

3.1. $pH = pK + \log \dfrac{[HCO_3^-]}{[CO_2]}$

   A. The term $[CO_2]$ can be replaced by $\alpha PaCO_2$
   B. The term $[HCO_3^-]$ refers to the standard bicarbonate
   C. The term pK is a constant and is not influenced by changes in pressure and temperature
   D. The ratio between $[HCO_3^-]$ and $[CO_2]$ determines the pH
   E. The equation is incorrect and should read
$$pH = pK + \log \dfrac{[CO_2]}{[HCO_3^-]}.$$

For each question 3.2 − 3.6, select the most appropriate diagnosis:

	pH	PCO$_2$	Standard Bicarbonate
3.2.	7.35	55	30
3.3.	7.55	47	40
3.4.	7.20	29	11
3.5.	7.35	28	15
3.6.	7.55	25	21

   A. Diabetic Ketoacidosis
   B. Partially compensated metabolic acidosis
   C. Partially compensated respiratory acidosis
   D. Overventilation during anaesthesia
   E. Pyloric stenosis.

Answers overleaf

3.1. A.

The equation is correct. α is the solubility coefficient. Thus $PaCO_2 = [CO_2]$. Standard bicarbonate is the plasma bicarbonate under the standard conditions: $PaCO_2 = 40$ mmHg, oxygenated, temperature $37°$ C. pH changes with the temperature and thus the ratio $[HCO_3]/[CO_2]$ cannot alone determine the pH.

3.2-C; 3.3-E; 3.4-A; 3.5-B; 3.6-D.

Acid base results are confusing partly because of the terminology and partly because the direction of two of the numerical scales is the reverse of the change they measure. A raised concentration of respiratory acid (respiratory acidosis) *is* represented by a high PCO_2, but a raised level of metabolic acids (measured when PCO_2 is normal — "standard" conditions) which could be represented by a high "standard" hydrogen ion concentration is instead represented by the reciprocal (a low standard bicarbonate), and a raised level of acidity (raised hydrogen ion concentration) is represented by a low negative logarithm. The object is to decide which of the two components (respiratory or metabolic) is changed in the same direction as the overall pH and is therefore responsible and which (if either) is changed in the opposite direction and is therefore compensating.

3.7. When the pH changes from 7.4 to 6.4, the hydrogen ion
     concentration changes by:

    A. Twofold increase
    B. Twofold decrease
    C. Tenfold increase
    D. Tenfold decrease
    E. Increasing by 1.414 times.

Answers overleaf

3.7. C

The concentration has changed from $10^{-7.4}$ to $10^{-6.4}$ mol/l. Thus the ratio between the two concentrations is $10^{(7.4-6.4)} = 10^1 = 10$.

3.8. The normal acidity of blood is:

    A. pH 7.4
    B. 400 nano mol/l hydrogen ion concentration
    C. 40 nano mol/l hydrogen ion concentration
    D. 0.000,40 mEq/l hydrogen ion
    E. 0.000,000,004 gram/l hydrogen ion.

Answers overleaf

3.8. A, C.

Insight into the meaning of pH can be obtained by deriving values personally. The few facts necessary are:

1. The meaning of "logarithm" can be understood if it is remembered that it is the same as the "power", thus $\log_{10}$ of 10,000 (10^4) is 4.0.
2. A tenfold increase in a number changes the log + 1.0
3. A twofold increase in a number changes the log + 0.3.
4. pH is the *negative* logarithm.

		log	pH	
1,000	mol/l	3	−3	⎫ Impossibly strong but
100	mol/l	2	−2	⎬ they make the idea
10	mol/l	1	−1	⎭ easier to grasp.
1	mol/l	0	0	
0.1	mol/l	−1	1	
0.01	mol/l	−2	2	
1 m mol/l		−3	3	⎫ i.e. for every thousand-
1 mic mol/l		−6	6	⎬ fold dilution, the loga-
1 nano mol/l		−9	9	⎭ rithm decreases by 3.
and ∴ { 10 nano mol/l		−8	8	
{ 100 nano mol/l		−7	7	

A table of clinical values can then be constructed:

ph values:	6.8	7.0	7.1	7.2	7.3	7.4	7.5	7.6	7.7	7.8	7.9	8.0
Insert the end points:		100										10
Step up from 10 in x 2 steps	160	←---	80	←---		40	←---		20	←---		10
Step down from 100 in ÷ 2 steps:		100			---→ 50			---→ 25			--→ 12.5	
Step ÷ 10 from 160	160	(as indicated) - -	-- - -	- - - -	- - - -	- - - -	- - -→			16		
Step up from 16 in x 2 stepa:				64	←----		32	←----		16		
This gives the complete logarithmic scale:	160	100	80	64	50	40	32	25	20	16	12.5	10

Normal acidity is (0.04) mic mol/l or 0.000,04 m mol/l

3.9. The following values expressed unconventionally may be found in a normal adult male:

    A. 5.5 million red cells/microlitre
    B. Haematocrit of 0.045
    C. 8 million white cells/cubic centimetre
    D. PaO_2 of 2 lb/in^2
    E. Haemoglobin of 14.5 g/l.

3.10. Of the following which has the highest concentration of sodium ions:

    A. Serum
    B. Sweat
    C. Blood
    D. Isotonic saline
    E. Gastric juice.

3.11. Found in thalassaemia
3.12. Treated successfully with reducing agents
3.13. Causes cyanosis unrelieved by methylene blue
3.14. Causes cyanosis which may be relieved by hyperbaric oxygen.

For each question 3.11, 3.12, 3.13, 3.14 select the best example only from:

    A. Methaemoglobin
    B. Foetal haemoglobin
    C. Sulphaemoglobin "S"
    D. Haemoglobin "S"
    E. Carboxyhaemoglobin.

Answers overleaf

3.9. A, C, D.

1 cubic metre (m^3) contains 1,000 cubic decametres (litres).
1 litre ($m^3 \times 10^{-3}$) contains 1,000 cubic centimetres (ml).
1 ml (cm^3 or $m^3 \times 10^{-6}$) contains 1,000 cubic millimetres (mic 1).
1 mic l is a cubic millimetre (mm^3 or $m^3 \times 10^{-9}$).
The normal blood values are 5.5 million red cells/mm^3, 8 thousand white cells/mm^3, a haemoglobin of 14.5 g/100 ml and a haematocrit of 45% which may be expressed as a fractional quantity — 0.45.

2lb/in^2 is approximately equal to the normal arterial oxygen tension (PaO_2) of 100 mmHg which is 100/760 of atmospheric pressure.

3.10. D.

Isotonic saline depends on sodium and chloride to achieve the tonicity which is achieved elsewhere in the body by many ions. Sweat is hypotonic until evaporation occurs. Active transport of sodium across cell membranes achieves 130 m mol/l in extracellular fluid. This is exceeded in the renal tubule where active transport of sodium from the ascending limb of the loop of Henle maintains the hypertonicity of the renal papillae.

3.11-B; 3.12-A; 3.13-C; 3.14 — no answer correct.

The reducing agents employed to treat methaemoglobinaemia include methylene blue and ascorbic acid. Carbon monoxide poisoning responds to hyperbaric oxygen treatment, but as carboxyhaemoglobin does not cause cyanosis there is no correct answer.

3.15. Plasma proteins may be determined by:

    A. Paper chromatography
    B. Polarography
    C. Precipitation methods
    D. Gas chromatography
    E. Electrophoresis.

3.16. Compound injection of sodium lactate B.P. (Ringer's Lactate, Hartmann's) contains:

    A. Sodium 112 mEq/l
    B. Chloride 131 mEq/l
    C. Bicarbonate 29 mEq/l
    D. Calcium 1.4 mEq/l
    E. Potassium 1.5 mEq/l.

3.17. Dextran 70:

    A. Has a molecular weight lower than albumin
    B. Can cause renal failure
    C. Is mostly cleared from the blood in four hours
    D. Cannot be mixed with dextrose
    E. Causes an osmotic diuresis.

3.18. Acute hyperkalaemia may be satisfactorily treated by the use of:

    A. Intravenous glucose and insulin
    B. Darrow's solution
    C. Ion exchange resins
    D. Intravenous thiazides
    E. Calcium gluconate 10%.

Answers overleaf

3.15. C, E.

Both paper and gas chromatography can determine amino-acids, sugars, etc. but cannot cope with large protein molecules. Precipitation methods are applicable to plasma protein and protein fraction estimations. By using wet paper to complete a circuit, each end dipped in electrolyte solutions, the charged protein molecules in a specimen placed on the paper will migrate at different *rates* along the paper strip. Therefore the proteins will migrate to different *lengths*, their presence being shown up as stripes by straining agents once the electrophoresis is complete.

3.16. All false.

The figures should be known because the contents are similar to normal serum levels, i.e. sodium 131 mEq/l, chloride 112 mEq/l, calcium 4.0 mEq/l, potassium 5.0 mEq/l.
Note there is no bicarbonate but 29 mEq/l of lactate bicarbonate could precipitate as chalk.

3.17. No correct answer.

The average molecular weight of Dextran 70 is 70,000 and like albumin (69,000) is unable to pass into glomerular filtrate, and is cleared from the blood slowly.
Dextrans of higher molecular weight can damage microcirculation and cause trouble with cross matching. Lower molecular weight dextrans pass into glomerular filtrate and can cause osmotic diuresis. Renal failure with Dextran 40 has been reported but controversial.

3.18. A, C, E.

Intravenous glucose and insulin facilitate the migration of potassium ions from the E.C.F. to the I.C.F. Ion exchange resins remain in the gut and exchange either calcium or sodium from their molecules for potassium. (The released sodium or calcium will be absorbed from the gut.) Calcium ions physiologically counteract the effect of potassium ions on the heart. Darrow's solution contains 36 mEq/l of potassium, 52 mEq/l of bicarbonate. Thiazides are contra-indicated because of risk of anuria or incipient renal failure associated with hyperkalaemia.

3.19. Which of the following organisms may be found contaminating disinfectants in hospital:

    A. Clostridium welchii
    B. Streptococcus viridans
    C. Eschericha coli
    D. Pseudomonas aeroginosa
    E. Staphylococcus pyogenes.

3.20. The following disinfectants are useful against Pseudomonas in a ventilator:

    A. Cetrimide solution B.P.C. (1%)
    B. Chlorhexidine hydrochloride in spirit
    C. Chlorhexidine hydrochloride in water
    D. Formaldehyde
    E. Ethylene oxide.

3.21. The following may be used during tests for pseudo-cholinesterase abnormality:

    A. Cinchocaine
    B. Sodium chloride
    C. Sodium fluoride
    D. Sodium bromide
    E. Bupivicaine.

3.22. The life of the adult human red cell is about:

    A.   5 days
    B. 20 days
    C. 50 days
    D. 120 days
    E. 180 days.

Answers overleaf

3.19. A, D.

Pseudomonas is the most likely contaminant. Tap water contains Clostridium welchii and solutions made up with tap water could be contaminated.

3.20. D, E.

Formaldehyde and ethylene oxide are satisfactory disinfectants against Pseudomonas in respiratory equipment, although stringent care is needed to remove all traces before use. Ethylene oxide is poinonous and explosive (3.3 to 80% in air) and easily absorbed by rubber. Chlorhexidine is normally made up in at least 7% by volume of ethyl alcohol or 4% by volume of isopropyl alcohol to try and prevent contamination with Pseudomonas. Cetrimide will grow Pseudomonas!

3.21. A, C.

Both cinchocaine (Dibucaine) and sodium fluoride inhibit normal pseudo-cholinesterase more than the atypical variety. Thus a high degree of inhibition (high Dibucaine number and high fluoride number) indicates normal pseudocholinesterase.

3.22. D.

The survival of normal red cells is about 120 days. However transfusion of blood (after 21 days storage) drops the maximum red cell survival to 100 days. The survival of other cells in the blood is considerably less. Neutrophils last about 2 days but their average stay in the circulation is only about 8 hours. They are very quickly destroyed in stored blood. Platelets exist in the circulation for 8—11 days. In stored blood they disintegrate in a few hours. When platelet-rich plasma or plasma concentrates have been produced they must be given within 6 hours of removal from donor. However the transfused platelet survival is only 2—4 days.

3.23. The total osmotic pressure of plasma is about:

    A. 22.4 atmospheres
    B.   6.5 atmospheres
    C.   2.5 atmospheres
    D. 650 mmHg
    E.   25 mmHg.

3.24. Cerebro-spinal fluid has a:

    A. Normal albumin content of 20 mg/100 ml
    B. PCO_2 higher than that of arterial blood
    C. Specific gravity of 1.040
    D. Raised globulin level in myotonia congenita
    E. Volume of about 60 ml. in the average-sized adult.

3.25. Which of the following are consistent with a diagnosis of acute renal tubular necrosis:

    A. Oliguria
    B. Polyuria
    C. Increased urine urea
    D. Hyperkalaemia
    E. Oedma.

3.26. Towards the end of the permitted period for storing A.C.D. (Bank) blood, which of the following levels would be expected:

    A. Na^+ 140 mEq/l.
    B. K^+ 8—9.5 mEq/l.
    C. Standard bicarbonate 32—35 mEq/l.
    D. PO_2 5—15 mmHg
    E. pH 5.2.

Answers overleaf

3.23. B.

One osmole dissolved in one litre exerts an osmotic pressure of 22.4 atmospheres. The normal osmolality of plasma is about 290 mOsm/Kg (= 6.5 atmos.), 25 mmHg is the oncotic (colloid osmotic) pressure due to the difference between the plasma oncotic pressure (about 35 mmHg) and the tissue oncotic pressure (about 10 mmHg).

3.24. A, B.

The specific gravity of C.S.F., is between 1.003 and 1.009. Normal albumin level is 20 mg/100 ml and the globulin level is 3 mg/100 ml. *Globulin* levels are raised in *chronic* infections. Albumin and globulin levels rise after spinal anaesthetics. The adult C.S.F., volume is 110—150 ml. C.S.F. PCO_2 has been found to be about 10 mmHg above that of arterial blood.

3.25. A, B, D, E.

Oliguria is the commonest finding of acute renal tubular necrosis. Complete anuria usually indicates organic obstruction. Polyuria is occasionally encountered in early tubular necrosis (e.g. with tetracyclines and methoxyflurane) and it is a feature of the recovery phase and commonly occurs between the 10th and 14th day. Hyperkalaemia tends to occur in oliguria. Urine urea concentration is low due to failure of tubular concentration.

3.26. A, D.

The sodium in banked blood is initially raised due to the Acid Citrate Dextrose and falls to about 140 mEq/l as it leaks into the cells in exchange for potassium. The potassium may reach 20 mEq/l. The standard bicarbonate is extremely low, reflecting the metabolic acidosis of anaerobic metabolism, and the pH approaches 6.5.

3.27. A serum osmolarity of 360 milliosmoles/litre is compatible with:

    A. Excessive secretion of anti-diuretic hormone
    B. Normal serum
    C. Uraemia
    D. Fresh water drowning
    E. Uncontrolled diabetes.

3.28. The aspartate transaminase is markedly raised:

    A. In hepatocellular liver disease
    B. In muscular dystrophy
    C. By breathing 5% carbon dioxide for five minutes
    D. After major cardiac surgery
    E. In hypovolaemia.

3.29. The alkaline phosphatase is elevated in:

    A. Paget's disease
    B. Carcinoma of the prostate confined to the prostate
    C. Osteosarcoma
    D. Obstructive jaundice
    E. Hyperthyroidism.

Answers overleaf

3.27. C, E.

Osmola*R*ity is a measure of the number of particles (ions and molecules) per lit*R*e of mixed solution (osmola*L*ity is a measure of the number per ki*L*ogram of water). Normal osmolarity is 275—295 mOsm/l. A.D.H. secretion and fresh water drowning tend to lower osmolarity. A high osmolarity could be caused by elevated levels of:

(1)	K^+, Ca^{++}, Mg^{++}.	A patient would die before such a marked elevation could be caused by these ions.
(2)	Urea, glucose, Na^+, water deprivation.	These are possible causes. While uraemic subjects are not thirsty, this symptom is very prominent with the others.
(3)	Therapeutic agents, e.g. mannitol and radiographic dyes, can raise osmolarity.	

3.28. A, D.

Aspartate transaminase is present in high concentration in heart and liver, and is released by damage to either. Some forms of muscle disease raise the creatine phosphokinase level (used to identify patients susceptible to malignant hyperpyrexia) markedly, while showing only a relatively small rise in transaminases.

3.29. A, C, D.

Alkaline phosphatase is an enzyme present in the osteoblasts of growing bone and in granulation tissue, liver, kidney and intestinal mucosa. Differentiation between liver and bone alkaline phosphatase is achieved by measuring 5-nucleotidase (raised in liver disease) or by electrophoresis. *Acid* phosphatase is elevated in carcinoma of the prostate. Osteosclerotic secondaries from the prostate may raise the *alkaline* phosphatase. Osteosarcoma is a complication of Paget's, often associated with a sudden, further rise in the alkaline phosphatase. Back pressure from obstructive jaundice causes the enzyme to be "regurgitated" into the blood. A rise in the liver alkaline phosphatase is a sensitive test of liver secondaries.

3.30. The following are used in the differential diagnosis of jaundice:

    A. Serum bilirubin
    B. Indirect van den Bergh reaction
    C. Direct van den Bergh reaction
    D. Prothrombin time
    E. Bleeding time.

3.31. A woman with group A Rh -ve blood:

    A. May be given Rh +ve blood after the menopause
    B. If pregnant with a baby with group B Rh +ve, is likely to have a healthy baby
    C. Should be given Anti D globulin after the delivery of her first baby
    D. May deliver a baby requiring exchange transfusion of Rh +ve blood
    E. Will not in her first pregnancy give birth to a child who becomes jaundiced.

3.32. Target cells are present in:

    A. Sickle-cell anaemia
    B. HbC disease
    C. Iron deficiency anaemia
    D. B_{12} deficiency
    E. Thalassaemia.

3.33. In a patient with untreated intestinal obstruction the most likely cause of death is:

    A. Water loss alone
    B. Sodium loss alone
    C. Sodium loss and water loss together
    D. Hypokalaemia
    E. Alkalosis.

Answers overleaf

3.30. A, B, C, D.

The level of the bilirubin depends on the cause of the jaundice (contrast the mild haemolytic jaundice of pernicious anaemia with the deep jaundice of common bile duct obstruction). An indirect van den Bergh reaction detects the bilirubin not yet conjugated by the liver (haemolysis). A direct reaction detects conjugated bilirubin (common bile duct obstruction, liver disease). The prothrombin time is prolonged in liver disease due to diminished synthesis of prothrombin and factors V, VII and X. The bleeding time detects vessel abnormalities (e.g. von Willebrand's disease).

3.31. B, C.

The most likely ways for a Rh -ve woman to be sensitised to Rh +ve blood are by transfusion (at any age) or at delivery of a Rh +ve child. When mother and child have ABO incompatibility as well, foetal red cells entering the maternal circulation are destroyed before causing production of Rh antibodies. Injection of Anti D shortly after delivery can similarly destroy foetal cells before the mother is sensitised. Exchange transfusion employs blood which will not be destroyed by maternal Anti D (i.e. Rh -ve blood). Newborn babies are frequently jaundiced for reasons other than Rh incompatibility.

3.32. A, B, C, E.

Target cells are red cells, larger than normal with a (relatively) small haemoglobin content and the appearance of rings (as in an archery target). They occur characteristically in Thalassaemia, with the microcytes in iron deficiency anaemia, in sickle cell anaemia and HbC disease.

3.33. D.

The direct myocardial effects of hypokalaemia considerably antecede the deleterious effects of the alternatives. Thus early attention to potassium replacement is essential in the management of such a patient which will, normally, include early surgery.

3.34. A serum sodium of 142 mM/l and a serum potassium of 6.2 mM/l is compatible with:

   A. Hypopituitarism
   B. Addison's disease
   C. Hypokalaemia
   D. Myxoedma
   E. The blood being taken from a bottle of stored (ACD) blood.

Answers overleaf

3.34. E.

Lack of endogenous steroids or ACTH (hypopituitarism or Addison's) would cause much lower Na^+. Hypokalaemia is incompatible by definition and there are no significant electrolyte changes in myxoedema. In stored blood potassium levels may considerably exceed the figure mentioned.

4. GENERAL PHYSIOLOGY

4.1. The following are involved in transmission at autonomic ganglia:

    A. Noradrenaline
    B. Acetyl choline
    C. G.A.B.A.
    D. Prostaglandins
    E. Adrenaline.

4.2. Symptoms of decompression sickness:

    A. May be pulmonary
    B. May be neurological
    C. May be cutaneous
    D. May be Skeletal
    E. Are inevitable following sudden decompression to normal conditions after prolonged exposure to two atmospheres absolute.

4.3. The secretion of aldosterone:

    A. Reduces sodium absorption in the proximal convoluted tubule
    B. Reduces sodium diffusion in the descending loop of Henle
    C. Increases sodium absorption in the distal convoluted tubule
    D. Reduces sodium absorption in the distal convoluted tubule
    E. Increases sodium absorption in the collecting tubule.

Answers overleaf

4.1. B.

The transmitter substance at *all* autonomic ganglia is acetyl choline. Noradrenaline is the transmitter substance at *post-ganglionic* neurones of the sympathetic system. Gamma amino butyric acid is an inhibitory transmitter at central nervous synapses. It is interesting to note that some anti-emetic drugs have a similar chemical structure to G.A.B.A. Adrenaline is mainly secreted by the adrenal medulla.

4.2. A, B, C, D.

The symptoms due to the formation of bubbles during decompression are known to divers, depending on the site, as the "chokes" (lungs), the "staggers" (neurological), the "itch" (skin) or the "bends" (skeletal). Decompression from 30 feet of water (2 atmospheres absolute) to surface does not cause decompression sickness.

4.3. C.

Aldosterone is secreted by the adrenal cortex in response to angiotensin II. It acts on the distal convoluted tubule to potentiate sodium absorption from the urine into the surrounding epithelial cells.

4.4. The secretion of anti-diuretic hormone (vasopressin):

   A. Decreases glomerular filtration rate
   B. Increases reabsorption of water in the proximal convoluted tubule
   C. Increases permeability of the distal convoluted tubule to water
   D. Increases permeability of the collecting tubule to water
   E. Increase osmolarity of urine.

4.5. The peripheral resistance of the circulation:

   A. Falls as the haematocrit falls
   B. Is greatly influenced by "tone" in the arterioles
   C. Rises with administration of dextran of molecular weight 70,000
   D. Is initially lowered by the administration of mannitol
   E. Is raised by hypercapnoea (Hypercarbia).

4.6. Inulin:

   A. Is cleared from the blood completely in a single passage through the kidney
   B. Is not reabsorbed from the glomerular filtrate
   C. Concentration in glomerular filtrate is equal to the plasma concentration
   D. Is secreted by kidney tubular cells
   E. Does not pass into the extravascular space.

Answers overleaf

4.4. C, D, E.

Antidiuretic hormone is secreted in the posterior pituitary under control of plasma osmolarity. It causes a breakdown in the "water-proofing" of the distal and collecting tubules. Water is passively reabsorbed and the urine becomes concentrated (osmolarity increased).

4.5. A, B, D.

The flow of blood through the blood vessels to a large extent obeys Poiseuille's law and resistance is proportional to viscosity. As the haematocrit increases so does the viscosity.

Alterations in tone of blood vessels causes an alteration in the radius (r) of the vessels. Flow is proportional to r^4. As the arterioles are the most muscular, they have the greatest capacity for changing the peripheral resistance.

Dextran 70 has a molecular weight of 70,000 and by increasing the plasma volume has the effect of diluting the red cell concentration, thus lowering the viscosity and therefore the peripheral resistance.

Mannitol is a high molecular weight substance which, when injected, causes fluid to move from the extravascular space into the blood vessels. Initially the haematocrit falls and so does the viscosity.

Hypercapnoea causes dilation of blood vessels.

4.6. B, C.

Inulin, a polymer of fructose (M.W. = 5,200) is used to measure the glomerular filtration rate. It is freely filterable and is not reabsorbed or secreted by tubules. Its low molecular weight allows it to pass into the extravascular space. All freely filterable substances have the same concentrate in the glomerular filtrate as in plasma. Although tubular reabsorption of water may alter the urine concentration of inulin, it does not alter the amount being excreted, and it can therefore be used to measure glomerular filtration rate.

4.7. The following ions may be concerned with the release of
acetyl choline at nerve terminals:

    A. K^+
    B. Mg^{++}
    C. Na^+
    D. Ca^+
    E. Ammonium.

4.8 In the normal subject the cerebral blood flow will be increased
by:

    A. An increase in the arterial PCO_2 to about 60 mmHg
    B. A head down posture
    C. An increase in systolic blood pressure from 110 mmHg
        to 130 mmHg
    D. Hyperventilation
    E. A rise in the arterial PO_2 .

4.9. Folic acid:

    A. Is involved in nucleic acid synthesis
    B. Is essential for D.N.A. synthesis
    C. Is essential for R.N.A. synthesis
    D. Can prevent subacute combined degeneration due to
        vitamin B_{12} deficiency
    E. Is specific therapy for the megaloblastic anaemia of
        vitamin B_{12} deficiency.

4.10 The blood oxygen dissociation curve is shifted to the left by:

    A. Low temperature
    B. Low haemoglobin levels
    C. Hypoxia
    D. Acidosis
    E. Alkalosis

Answers overleaf

4.7. B, D.

Calcium is essential for the release of acetyl choline at the synaptic junction whereas magnesium appears to antagonize this release.

4.8. A.

Changes of posture and moderate alteration in blood pressure do not affect the cerebral blood flow. In contrast the flow is sensitive to small changes in arterial gas tensions. Thus, either a rise in arterial PCO_2 or a fall in arterial PO_2 cause an increase in cerebral blood flow.

4.9. A, B, E.

Folic acid (pteroylglutamic acid) and vitamin B_{12} are both required for erythropoiesis and C.N.S. function. Folic acid must not be used alone to treat patients with pernicious anaemia (B_{12} deficiency) because subacute combined degeneration of the spinal cord may be precipitated even though the anaemia is (at least temporarily) corrected.

4.10. A, E.

The blood oxygen dissociation curve is independent of haemoglobin concentration (although haemoglobin concentration does of course influence blood's oxygen content). It is helpful to picture actively metabolizing muscle producing *acid*, CO_2 and *heat*. All of these shift the curve to the right and therefore help to dissociate oxygen from haemoglobin.

4.11. In a normal heart:

A. The resting potential on the outside of a muscle cell is +80 to 90 mV
B. The time between spontaneous firing of the sino-atrial node and the contraction of the atria is the PR interval
C. The sino-atrial node is located where the right atrial wall joins the superior vena cava
D. The sino-atrial node resting potential is more than 90 mV
E. The QRS complex should not be longer than 0.12 sec.

4.12. Which of the following can break down noradrenaline:

A. Catechol-o-methyl transferase
B. Monomine oxidase
C. Serum aspartate transaminase
D. Serum hydroxy butyric acid
E. Dopamine β-hydroxylase.

4.13. Pancreatic secretions:

A. Increase conversion of galactose to glucose
B. Increase fat absorption
C. Decrease liver glycogen
D. Decrease sucrose absorption
E. Increase hexamethonium's ganglion-blocking action.

4.14. The rate of emptying of the stomach is decreased by:

A. Acid in duodenum
B. Raised osmolarity of duodenal contents
C. Fat in duodenum
D. Atropine injection
E. Fear.

Answers overleaf

4.11. A, C, E.

The time between spontaneous firing of the sino-atrial node and ventricular contraction is the PR interval. There is no steady resting potential for the sino-atrial node. It is about 80 mV maximum before reducing towards the critical value required for triggering. The QRS complex is the time taken for the stimulus to spread throughout the ventricles and normally is about 0.11 sec.

4.12. A, B.

Circulating noradrenaline and adrenaline are methylated to biologically inactive substances by catechol-o-methyl transferase (C.O.M.T.). In adrenergic nerve endings some of the noradrenaline is constantly being destroyed by monoamine oxidase. Serum aspartate transaminase and serum hydroxy butyric acid are enzymes found in large amounts in the liver and do not affect noradrenaline. Dopamine β-hydroxylase is an enzyme required to change dopamine into noradrenaline.

4.13. B, C.

Pancreatic secretions include insulin and glucagon as well as the exocrine secretion of pancreatic juice. Glucagon raises blood sugar by mobilizing liver glycogen. Pancreatic amylase breaks down polysaccharides (i.e. starches) to tri- and di-saccharides. Sucrose is a disaccharide and has to be broken down into its constituent monosaccharides prior to absorption. Lipases break down fats for absorption as fatty acids and glycerol. One of the signs of chronic pancreatitis is fatty, smelly stools. Hexamethonium decreases the secretion of pancreatic juice.

4.14. A, C, D, E.

The enterogastric reflex is a neurally mediated reflex causing decrease in gastric mobility. Fats, products of protein digestion and hydrogen ions entering the duodenum, as well as fear and duodenal distension, all initiate this reflex by causing the release of secretin into the circulation which inhibits gastric mobility and secretion. Atropine decreases the tone and peristalsis of the gut.

4.15. Carbohydrate is the sole source of energy in:

    A. Myocardium
    B. Skeletal muscle
    C. Brain
    D. Kidney
    E. Adipose tissue.

Answers overleaf

4.15. C.

Brain metabolism depends on a supply of glucose because the blood/brain barrier prevents other substrates passing in quantities sufficient to maintain normal metabolic rates. In contrast, the heart can metabolize glucose, lactate, pyruvate, ketones, fatty acids and fat.

5. MEDICINE

5.1. In sickle cell disease:

    A. The haemoglobin has an abnormality of the beta-poly-
        peptide chains
    B. The haemoglobin becomes less soluble when in the re-
        duced form
    C. The haemoglobin is 90—95% of the foetal type
    D. The commonest form of crisis is independent of tactoid
        formation
    E. Alkalosis may be hazardous because it shifts the oxygen
        dissociation curve to the left.

5.2. Large quantities of urine may be excreted due to:

    A. Posterior pituitary damage
    B. Therapy with tolbutamide
    C. Renal failure
    D. Gout
    E. Thyrotoxicosis.

5.3. In myasthenia gravis:

    A. Thyrotoxicosis is an associated condition
    B. Edrophonium improves muscle power
    C. Anxiety impairs muscle power
    D. Following thymectomy, the improvement in muscle
        power occurs within 7–10 days in most cases
    E. Demyelination occurs in peripheral nerves.

Answers overleaf

5.1. A, B, E.

The sixth position on the beta-polypeptide chain, normally occupied by glutamic acid, is substituted by valine. The alpha-chains are normal. In sickle cell anaemia 5—10% of the haemoglobin present is of the foetal type.

The sickling phenomenon is related to tactoid formation. While alkalosis is "anti-sickling", it confers the hazard of shifting the oxygen dissociation curve to the left which inhibits oxygen release to the tissues. (Acidosis, however, is more hazardous as it is directly sickle-provoking.)

5.2. A, C.

A.D.H. secretion may be inhibited by pituitary damage. While renal failure generally leads to oliguria and anuria, a lack of concentrating power in early stages will lead to a high output failure.

5.3. A, B, C.

A small percentage of myasthenics also have thyrotoxicosis. Anticholinesterases improve power, edrophonium being a useful diagnostic test. Psychic trauma may precipitate a myasthenic crisis. Improvement in muscle power after thymectomy may not be noticed for months; early benefit is rare.

5.4. Myxoedma may present with:

    A. Carpel tunnel syndrome
    B. Hallucinations
    C. Cardiomegaly
    D. Raised alkaline phosphatases
    E. Coma.

5.5. Hyperparathyroidism may present with:

    A. Osteitis fibrosa
    B. Renal stones
    C. Tetany
    D. Peptic ulceration
    E. Osteoporosis.

5.6. Finger clubbing is diagnostically associated with:

    A. Ulcerative colitis
    B. Chronic bronchitis
    C. Meig's syndrome
    D. Blue sclerotics
    E. Subungual haemorrhages.

Answers overleaf

5.4. A, B, C, E.

Myxoedma has diverse presentations. The serum cholesterol is often raised. The patient may present (or be referred) to any hospital department, e.g.

Medicine (myocardial ischaemia on E.C.G., hypertension, anaemia)
Surgery (obstruction, constipation, goitre)
Gynaecology (amenorrhoea)
Psychiatry (phychosis)
Dermatology (rough, scaly skin)
Orthopaedics (carpel tunnel syndrome)
E.N.T. (hoarse voice)
Ophthalmic (exophthalmos post-thyroidectomy)
Physical medicine ("rheumatism")
Neurology (coma).

5.5. A, B, D.

Hypercalcaemia is the feature and causes osteitis fibrosa (but not osteoporosis), renal stones and gastro-intestinal problems. Tetany is related to a reduction in ionized calcium which is common in hypoparathyroidism (occasionally seen as a post-operative complication following thyroidectomy). Voluntary hyperventilation will usually produce tetany due to the respiratory alkalosis diminishing the ionized/unionized calcium ratio.

5.6. A, E.

Clubbing is found in certain chronic gut disorders — steatorrhea, ulcerative colitis, Crohn's disease. While chronic suppurative pulmonary conditions classically produce clubbing, bronchitis does not. Meig's syndrome is found with ovarian carcinoma and blue sclera in fragilitas ossium; neither of these conditions show clubbing. Finger clubbing joins with splinter (subungual) haemorrhages and Osler's nodes as diagnostically supportive of subacute bacterial endocarditis.

5.7. Ankylosing spondylitis has association with:

- A. Positive S.C.A.T. and latex tests
- B. Plantar fasciitis
- C. Iritis
- D. Aortic incompetance
- E. Psoriasis.

5.8. The following diseases are more common in men than women:

- A. Rheumatoid arthritis
- B. Polycythaemia rubra vera
- C. Von Willebrand's disease
- D. Addison's disease
- E. Dystrophia myotonica.

5.9. In haemophilia:

- A. The bleeding time is prolonged
- B. Epistaxis is common
- C. Even severe forms do not manifest before the second year of life
- D. There is a deficiency of factor VII
- E. Cryoprecipitate from stored blood will arrest haemorrhage.

5.10. Paroxysmal atrial tachycardia:

- A. May be arrested by carotid sinus massage
- B. Is an ideal indication for lignocaine therapy
- C. Occurs not infrequently in aged thyrotoxicosis
- D. Responds favourably to β-adrenergic blockers
- E. Is readily distinguished from ventricular tachycardia by E.C.G.

Answers overleaf

5.7. B, C, D.

Plantar fasciitis, iritis and aoritis are associated conditions. The R.A. and latex tests are negative. Psoriotic arthropathies are peripheral in character.

5.8. B.

Rheumatoid arthritis is commoner in women. The last three conditions do not show significant sexual discrimination. (Nevertheless, frontal baldness and gonadal atrophy in men seem to be well remembered signs of dystrophia myotonica.)

5.9. None correct

Because haemophilia shows a coagulative defect only, bleeding time is normal and epistaxis is not a common feature as it is in, e.g. thrombocytopenia. The missing factor is internationally known as factor VIII and in severe deficiency the condition may arise soon after the first month, although the early neonate shows immunity. Blood stored at $4°C$ quickly loses the sensitive factor VIII; thus cryoprecipitate must be isolated from fresh blood.

5.10. A, C, D.

Carotid massage frequently aborts the tachycardia. Such a dysrhythmia may be the presenting feature of thyrotoxicosis in the elderly. Unlike ventricular tachycardia, the atrial variety responds well, not to lignocaine treatment, but to β-blocking agents. The fast rate makes identification of discrete P waves difficult and, if the tachycardia is persistent, E.C.G. patterns may defy diagnosis.

Medicine

5.11. A patient in acute left ventricular failure will safely benefit in the emergency situation from:

A. High oxygen concentrations
B. Subcutaneous adrenaline to relieve bronchospasm
C. Venous tourniquets applied to the limbs
D. Intravenous digitalization
E. Intravenous frusemide.

5.12. Early features of an incompatible blood transfusion in a conscious patient are:

A. Lumbar pain
B. Jaundice
C. Nausea
D. Paraesthesia in limbs
E. Dyspnoea.

5.13. A heart is arrested in diastole. Possible causes are:

A. Hypercalcaemia
B. Hyperkalaemia
C. Acidosis
D. Digitalis overdose
E. Hypothermia.

Answers overleaf

5.11. A, C, E.

This is not an occasion demanding controlled low concentration oxygen administration. Adrenaline might be dangerous to a hypoxic and possibly damaged myocardium. Rapid digitalization may be unsafe if the condition has been precipitated by an infarct. Both venous tourniquets and diuresis will safely reduce the central venous return and effectively reduce the input load on the left ventricle.

5.12. A, C, D, E.

Jaundice occurs relatively late in common with haemoglobin-aemia, haemoglobinuria and oliguria. Lumbar and precordial pain, nausea, dyspnoea, fullness in the head, tingling of the limbs are all early features in the conscious patient. Under anaesthesia — hypotension, tachycardia, venous oozing (due to consumptive coagulopathy) and cyanosis are the usual indications of incompatibility.

5.13. B, C, E.

Calcium increases myocardial contraction force and increases myocardial excitability. Hyperkalaemia slows conduction time and inhibits the myocardium leading to ventricular standstill. Acidosis decreases myocardial contractility and also releases potassium from within the cell which further weakens the heart. While therapeutic digitalis classically slows the heart, severe digitalis toxicity leads to ventricular tachycardia, dysrhythmia and subsequently to ventricular fibrillation. Hypothermia in the moderate range may cause cardiac arrest from ventricular fibrillation, but levels below 15°C may lead to diastolic arrest.

6. PHARMACOLOGY

6.1. Diminished vascularity of the toxic goitre may be satisfactorily achieved with:

    A. Methyl-thiouracil
    B. Carbimazole
    C. Lugol's iodine
    D. Potassium iodide
    E. Radio-iodine, I^{131}.

6.2. A highly ionized drug:

    A. Is well absorbed from the intestine
    B. Is excreted mainly in the kidney
    C. Crosses the placental barrier easily
    D. Is reabsorbed from the renal tubule
    E. Is highly protein bound.

6.3. Digoxin toxicity may be treated with:

    A. Practolol
    B. Lignocaine
    C. Intravenous potassium
    D. Phenytoin
    E. Atropine.

Answers overleaf

6.1. C, D.

Potassium iodide is the active ingredient of Lugol's iodine given pre-operatively to diminish vascularity of the toxic goitre. Although antithyroid drugs, such as methyl-thiouracil and carbimazole, inhibit the formation of thyroid hormone by inhibiting the binding of iodine they increase the vascularity. I^{131} does not influence vascularity; in hyperthyroidism tracer doses are used diagnostically and larger doses therapeutically.

6.2. B.

Small ions are able to pass through the pores between cells, but for a drug to cross a cell membrane (e.g. intestine, placenta) it must be lipid soluble and therefore unionized. However, certain small ions may in addition be *actively* transported across cell membranes. It is of interest that antacids will increase the ionization of acids (e.g. aspirin) thus hindering their absorption. Although it is the ionized fraction of a drug that may become protein bound, the degree of protein binding is determined by the pK, the pH and the quantity of the protein present.

6.3. A, B, C, D.

Cardiac dysrhythmias may be treated with β_1 blockers, phenytoin, lignocaine and quinidine, but these drugs should be used with extreme caution in atrioventricular block as they are cardiac depressants. Potassium is usually required although it must be administered with extreme caution especially when given intravenously. The vagal bradycardia caused by digitalis does respond to atropine, but the serious toxic effect is on atrioventricular conductivity and here atropine is ineffective.

6.4. Duration of action of barbiturates is decreased by:

    A. Substitution of sulphur for oxygen in the 2 position of the ring
    B. Methylation in the 1 or 3 position of the ring
    C. Formation of sodium salts
    D. Branching of carbon chain 5 position of the ring
    E. Desaturation of carbon chain in 5 position of the ring

6.5 Which of the following drugs are mono-amine oxidase inhibitors:

    A. Hydroxyzine
    B. Deserpidine
    C. Amitriptyline
    D. Pargyline
    E. Perphenazine.

6.6. The initial actions of intra-venous mannitol are:

    A. Increased blood viscosity
    B. Increased haematocrit
    C. Expansion of the blood volume
    D. Haemolysis
    E. Reduction in the extracellular volume.

Answers overleaf

6.4. A, B, D, E.

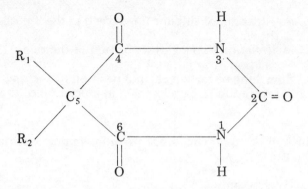

The duration of action is decreased by substitution of sulphur for oxygen at the 2 position and by substitution of a methyl group for the nitrogen in position 1 or 3. Branching and desaturation of the chains in position 5 lead to increased potency and decreased duration of action. Alkyl groups on both nitrogen atoms, or, on C_5 if longer than 6 carbon atoms, produce convulsant properties. Phenyl groups on C_5 are associated with anticonvulsant properties.

6.5. D.

Hydroxyzine is a non-phenothiazine tranquillizer and antihistaminic. Deserpidine is a rauwolfia alkaloid with fewer side effects than reserpine but less constant in its tranquillizing action. Amitriptyline is a tricyclic antidepressant. Pargyline is a M.A.O.I. Perphenazine is a phenothiazine derivative.

6.6. C.

Mannitol draws water into the plasma from the red cell, from the interstitial fluid and from other cells and there is consequently an initial blood volume expansion. The viscosity and haematocrit fall as the blood volume rises. The total extracellular volume rises initially.

6.7. Which of the following agents have bronchodilator actions:

    A. Pethidine
    B. Morphine
    C. Ether
    D. Pancuronium
    E. Helium.

Answers overleaf

6.7. A, C.

Pethidine will relax bronchial muscle whereas morphine may actually cause bronchoconstriction. Ether causes bronchodilatation and is appropriately used in asthmatics. Pancuronium is said to have no action on bronchial musculature, although one case of bronchospasm has already been reported. Helium is used to reduce the density of inspired gases to lessen resistance caused by turbulent flow.

6.8. The following deplete noradrenaline at the post-ganglionic nerve terminals:

    A. Bretylium
    B. Guanethidine
    C. Imipramine
    D. Reserpine
    E. Monoamine oxidase inhibitors.

Answers overleaf

Pharmacology

6.8. B, C, D.

Noradrenaline is released from the mobile pool II by an action potential developed at the nerve terminal. Bretylium blocks this release, whereas guanethidine causes active release from this pool, leading to eventual depletion. Imipramine blocks the reuptake of noradrenaline from the E.C.F. into mobile pool I. The extracellular noradrenaline is metabolized by catechol-o-methyl transferase. Reserpine blocks the reuptake of noradrenaline from the cytoplasmic pool (I) into the intragranular pool II and this cytoplasmic noradrenaline is metabolized by monoamine oxidase, leading to depletion. Inhibitors of this enzyme not only inhibit this metabolic pathway, but also have an action similar to bretylium.

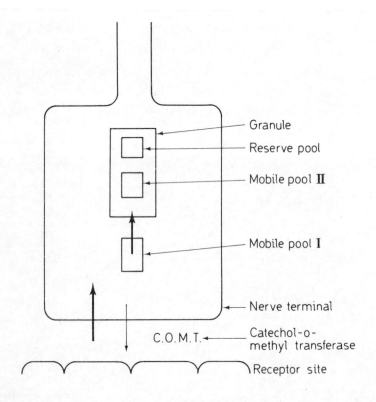

6.9. The following have a bronchoconstrictive action:

    A. Methoxamine
    B. Oxprenolol
    C. Practolol
    D. Nitrous oxide
    E. Propranolol.

6.10. Which of the following agents cross the blood/brain barrier:

    A. Tubocurarine
    B. Hexamethonium
    C. Lignocaine
    D. Hyoscine hydrobromide
    E. Sulphadiazine.

6.11. Isoprenaline:

    A. Inhibits the release of histamine
    B. Can be used sublingually
    C. May make ventilation/perfusion inequality worse
    D. Causes bradycardia
    E. Is a bronchodilator.

6.12. The following have sedative properties:

    A. Phenytoin
    B. Reserpine
    C. Chlorothiazide
    D. Methyldopa
    E. Lithium chloride.

Answers overleaf

6.9. B, E.

Oxprenolol and Propranolol both have β_1 and β_2 adrenergic blocking activity and can cause dangerous bronchoconstriction in asthmatics. Practolol's activity is said to be confined to the heart (β_1) although some β_2 activity cannot be excluded.

6.10. C, D, E.

For a drug to cross the blood/brain barrier it must be lipid soluble. Highly ionized drugs such as hexamethonium (a quaternary ammonium compound) do not, therefore, readily cross this hypothetical barrier.

Lignocaine and hyoscine have a central depressant action. All sulphonamides cross the blood/brain barrier but sulphadiazine crosses in amounts sufficient to be clinically effective.

6.11. A, B, C, E.

Isoprenaline stimulates all β-adrenergic receptors but has a minimal action on the α-receptors. It inhibits the release of histamine in sensitized human lungs to an even greater extent than salbutamol or disodium cromoglycate. Although it is used sublingually absorption is erratic and there is a risk of buccal ulceration.

6.12. B.

Phenytoin is a non-sedative anti-convulsant. Lithium chloride is unlike other anti-psychotic drugs in that it has no sedative properties.

6.13. The action of tubocurarine may be enhanced in:

    A. Liver failure
    B. Renal failure
    C. Streptomycin administration
    D. Hypothermia
    E. Hypercarbia.

6.14. Drugs which have an inhibitory effect on smooth muscle in the gut include:

    A. Amitriptyline
    B. Propantheline
    C. Atropine
    D. Hyoscine
    E. Pargyline.

6.15. These drugs have β-adrenergic blocking properties:

    A. Phenoxybenzamine
    B. Propranolol
    C. Oxprenolol
    D. Practolol
    E. Phentolamine.

6.16. A 2.5% solution of thiopentone:

    A. Has a pH of 6.8
    B. Is less than 50% protein bound when given intravenously
    C. Is metabolized at a rate of 20% per hour
    D. Is an analgesic
    E. Is a sulphur analogue of pentobarbitone.

Answers overleaf

6.13. C, E.

The low albumin level in hepatic failure is associated with a raised globulin level with increased protein binding of tubocurarine; also, cholinesterase production is impaired. Hence larger doses are required. The liver eliminates more tubocurarine in the bile in renal failure. Streptomycin has a curare-like action. Hypothermia reduces curarization. Hypercarbia potentiates and prolongs curarization.

6.14. A, B, C, D.

Propantheline, atropine and hyoscine are parasympathetic antagonists; amitriptyline and pargyline are antidepressants. Amitriptyline has atropine-like side effects, but pargyline (an M.A.O. inhibitor) does not.

6.15. B, C, D.

Phenoxybenzamine and phentolamine are α-adrenergic blocking agents, the action of the former lasting several days.
Propranolol is a β_1 and β_2-blocking agent, whereas practolol and oxprenolol have predominately β_1-blocking actions (cardiac).

6.16. C, E.

Thiopentone is the sulphur analogue of pentobarbitone and is very alkaline (pH 10.6). It is not an analgesic (anti-analgesic properties have been reported). It is metabolized at 16—24% per hour and is highly protein bound.

6.17. The following have analgesic properties:

    A. Droperidol
    B. Fentanyl
    C. Pentazocine
    D. Phenelzine
    E. Promethazine.

6.18. When ganglion-blocking hypotensive agents are used
6.19. When ecothiopate (Phospholine) eye drops are used
6.20. In severe liver disease
6.21. In myasthenia gravis

    For the above questions select the applicable answers from:

    A. Tubocurarine is potentiated
    B. Tubocurarine is antagonized
    C. Suxamethonium is potentiated
    D. Suxamethonium is antagonized
    E. Gallamine is potentiated.

6.22. Which of the following doses of cocaine might properly be used for a 70 kgm man aged 50 and in good health:

    A. 1 gram
    B. 10 ml of 1% solution
    C. 2 ml of 20% solution
    D. 1 ml of 10% solution
    E. 5 ml of 4.0% solution.

Answers overleaf

6.17. B, C.

Fentanyl and pentazocine are strong analgesics. Droperidol is a "tranquillizer" often combined with fentanyl in neuroleptanalgesia. Phenelzine is a monoamine oxidase inhibitor. Promethazine is an antihistamine used for its atropine-like and sedative actions in premedication and has been associated with "antanalgesia".

6.18-A, E; 6.19-B, C; 6.20-B, C; 6.21-A, D, E.

Ganglionic blockers have some competitive neuromuscular blocking action. The long-acting anti-cholinesterase ecothiopate has the same effect as low plasma cholinesterase due to severe liver disease. Additionally in liver disease, the albumin/globulin ratio is reversed, permitting high globulin binding of tubocurarine and thus affecting antagonism. Myasthenics behave as though partially curarized and are resistant to suxamethonium.

6.22. D, E.

The maximum safe dose of cocaine is about 3 mg/kg although the recommended dose for 10% cocaine is only 1.0 ml. It is toxic when injected but is a good surface anaesthetic when used in concentrations between 4.0 and 20%.

6.23. Lignocaine
6.24. Prilocaine
6.25. Cocaine
6.26. Amethocaine
6.27. Bupivicaine.

For questions 6.23 –6.27 select the appropriate statements from:

A. Inhibits bacteriostatic action of the sulphonamides
B. Has a vasoconstrictive action
C. Has the longest duration of effect
D. Is a satisfactory surface analgesic for mucous membranes
E. Hydrolyzed by pseudocholinesterase.

6.28. Which of the following are absorbed from the alimentary tract:

A. Ergot
B. Oxytocin
C. Atropine
D. Pentamethonium
E. Adrenaline.

6.29. Which of the following occur naturally:

A. Morphine
B. Heroin
C. Codeine
D. Ouabaine
E. Thebaine.

Answers overleaf

6.23-D; 6.24-D; 6.25-B, D; 6.26-A, D, E; 6.27-C, D.

A breakdown product of amethocaine — P.A.B.A. (para-amino benzoic acid) — competes with sulphonamides for entry into cells. Cocaine is powerfully vasoconstrictor. Bupivicaine (Marcaine) has the longest duration effect, making it especially suitable for epidurals. All five are surface analgesics. Amethocaine, like procaine, is hydrolyzed by pseudocholinesterase.

6.28. A, B, C.

Ergot is readily absorbed from the gastro-intestinal tract. (It was a cause of gangrene in people eating ergot-infested rye.) Oxytocin, which has a similar action on the uterus, can be absorbed from the buccal membrane, but the absorption is irregular. Atropine is readily absorbed (remember poisoning from ingesting "Deadly Nightshade"). Pentamethonium is a highly ionized quaternary ammonium compound and is therefore not absorbed from the alimentary tract and adrenaline is rapidly metabolized by monoamine oxidases in the gut.

6.29. A, C, D, E.

Morphine, codeine, thebaine (with papaverine and narcotine) are constituents of papaveratum (Omnopon) whereas heroin is synthesized from morphine. Ouabaine is a naturally occurring cardiac glycoside obtained from Strophanthus gratus seeds.

6.30. Which of the following are true statements:

A. Digitalis prolongs the refractory period of ventricular muscle
B. Lignocaine has a negative inotropic effect on the heart
C. Atropine slows the ventricular rate in atrial fibrillation
D. Propranolol increases the heart rate in sinus rhythm
E. Ventricular ectopic beats may be abolished by procaine.

6.31. Which of the following potentiate the action of tubocurarine:

A. Low serum K^+
B. High serum H^+
C. Low Ca^{++}
D. Renal acidosis
E. Myasthenic syndrome.

6.32. Which of the following are competitive antagonists:

A. Morphine and nalorphine
B. Histamine and perphenazine
C. Phenobarbitone and bemegride
D. Acetyl choline and gallamine
E. Hexamethonium and methoxamine.

Answers overleaf

6.30. B, E.

Digitalis has a positive inotropic action, being excitant to cardiac muscle. The rate of fibrillation may increase. However it slows conduction of impulses in the bundle of His and may thus slow the ventricular rate.

Lignocaine, propranolol and procaine have a membrane-stabilizing action giving rise to negative inotropic actions and control of ventricular ectopics. Their β-adrenergic blocking action, particularly that of propranolol, slows the heart rate so that myocardial work and cardiac output are reduced.

Atropine blocks the vagal action on the heart and therefore causes a rise in pulse rate, although an initial slowing, due to its central stimulatory action, may be detected.

6.31. A, B, C, D, E.

Acidaemia, whether of respiratory or renal origin, poteniates the action of tubocurarine, possibly by altering the degree of ionization and protein binding leading to higher plasma levels.

Hypokalaemia is associated with muscle weakness and even paralysis, and this is caused by a raising of the membrane potential.

In normal neuromuscular transmission there is a balance between calcium and magnesium ions, the latter tending to give a neuromuscular block. It follows that hypocalcaemia would cause this action of magnesium to predominate.

6.32. A, B, D.

Competitive antagonists are drugs which compete for the same receptors in the body. In contrast physiological antagonists counteract the action of the agonist in the tissue or organ affected. Thus bemegride, an analeptic, may be used to counteract the depressant action of barbiturates by its stimulating action. Similarly, the α-sympathomimetic amine methoxamine will counteract the peripheral vasodilatation caused by the ganglion-blocking agent, hexamethonium.

6.33. Which of the following are true:

    A. Atropine has a similar effect on the pulse rate as hyoscine

    B. Atropine reverses some of the effects of morphine

    C. Promethazine has an "atropine-like" action

    D. Morphine relieves pulmonary oedema

    E. Pethidine has local anaesthetic properties.

6.34. A neuromuscular agent causes momentary contraction of the tibialis anterior muscle of the cat. You would expect:

    A. Reversibility with neostigmine

    B. In incomplete paralysis there would be a sustained response to a tetanic stimulus

    C. The development of dual block with repeated use

    D. Prolonged action after poisoning with organophosphates

    E. Tachycardia following repeated doses.

6.35. Prostaglandin $F_2\alpha$:

    A. Is a naturally occurring polypeptide

    B. Causes bronchodilatation

    C. Causes contraction of the gravid uterus

    D. Lowers the blood pressure

    E. Has effects which are inhibited by aspirin.

Answers overleaf

6.33. B, C, D, E.

Although some doses of atropine can cause transient bradycardia, the normal response is marked tachycardia, particularly
in slow resting rates. Hyoscine has only minor effects on the
heart.

Atropine reverses some actions of morphine, particularly those
on the eye and gut. In common with atropine the phenothiazines
are vagolytic, antiemetic and have local anaesthetic properties.

The mechanism of the action of morphine in pulmonary
oedema is obscure, but may be due to improved cardiovascular
activity.

6.34. B, C, D.

The characteristics expected would be those of a depolarizing
muscle relaxant. Repeated use would allow the development of a
dual block. Organophosphates and neostigmine both prevent
hydrolysis of suxamethonium by pseudocholinesterase. The
vagal effects would tend to produce bradycardia.

6.35. C, E.

Prostaglandins (PGs) are derived from the fatty acid prostanoic
acid. The PG-Es cause bronchodilatation whereas the PG-Fs
cause bronchoconstriction. Asthma in some patients may be due
to an imbalance between these two series. Because PGs are
rapidly inactivated in the lungs, they cannot be given system-
ically. Aspirin and other antipyretic analgesics inhibit prostaglandin synthetase.

6.36. Morphine:

    A. Reduces sensory nerve conduction
    B. Stimulates the oculomotor nuclei
    C. Causes respiratory acidosis
    D. Is a diuretic
    E. Is used as an anaesthetic in cardiac-bypass surgery.

6.37. Noradrenaline slows the heart by:

    A. Direct action on the sino-atrial node
    B. Slowing atrio-ventricular conduction
    C. Decreasing venous return
    D. Increasing cardiac output
    E. Myocardial depression.

6.38. The following drugs uncouple oxidative phosphorylation:

    A. Barbiturates
    B. Salicylates
    C. Atropine
    D. Organophosphates
    E. Cyanide.

Answers overleaf

6.36. B, C, E.

Morphine is a central depressant, but does stimulate the Edinger-Westphal nucleus giving rise to constriction of the pupil. Its analgesic action is mainly due to a central alteration in reaction to pain.

Depression of the respiratory centre causes a respiratory acidosis.

Morphine causes increased ureteric tone and the detrusor tone of the bladder is increased. While this may lead to a sense of urgency, morphine, like other narcotic analgesics, has a mild anti-diuretic action. Morphine is usefully employed as the sole anaesthetic during open heart surgery, because it has no myocardial depressant effects in contrast with most other anaesthetics. (A positive inotropic action has been ascribed to it by some workers.)

6.37. None correct.

Noradrenaline has predominantly α-sympathomimetic effects. The heart rate is slowed through the action of raised blood pressure on the baroceptors. The cardiac output remains constant, although there is increased irritability and contractility of the myocardium.

6.38. A, B, E.

Barbiturates, salicylates and cyanide all uncouple oxidative phosphorylation. In consequence, a number of A.T.P.-dependent reactions are inhibited. The resulting metabolic deficiency may cause increased oxygen requirement and a pyretic effect as the energy which would be used to convert A.D.P. to A.T.P. is dissipated as heat.

6.39. Chlorpromazine is:

   A. A weak anti-histamine
   B. An α-adrenergic blocker
   C. A major tranquillizer
   D. A cause of Parkinsonism
   E. A curare antagonist.

6.40. Methaemoglobinaemia can result from deliberate or
      accidental exposure to:

   A. Phenacetin
   B. Methylene blue
   C. Prilocaine
   D. Paracetamol
   E. Paraldehyde.

6.41. The following drugs are metabolized by serum butyryl
      cholinesterase:

   A. Pethidine
   B. Morphine
   C. Bupivicaine
   D. Lignocaine
   E. Propanidid.

6.42. The following drugs have local anaesthetic properties:

   A. Carbimazole
   B. Morphine
   C. Pethidine
   D. Propranolol
   E. Gallamine.

Answers overleaf

6.39. A, B, C, D.

Chlorpromazine is a phenothiazine and like promethazine is an antihistamine. The actions of chlorpromazine on the sympathetic nervous system are complex. In vitro it has an α-adrenergic blocking action. In vivo this action may be masked. Chlorpromazine may potentiate the action of competitive neuromuscular blocking agents.

6.40. A, C.

Methaemoglinaemia is caused when a drug oxidizes the ferrous ion (Fe^{++}) to the ferric ion (Fe^{+++}). Phenacetin can cause methaemoglobinaemia whereas its breakdown product, paracetamol, does not. Prilocaine is the only local anaesthetic reported to produce methaemoglobinaemia. Methylene blue (like ascorbic acid) is a reducing agent suitable for treating methaemoglobinaemia.

6.41. E.

This is the familiar "pseudocholinesterase". Cinchocaine (Dibucaine) inhibits this enzyme. Propanidid is inactivated by esterases which split its ester bond.

6.42. C, D.

Carbimazole is only available as tablets. Morphine and gallamine have no local anaesthetic activity. Pethidine has potent local analgesic activity but because of its other actions is not used for this action.

Propranolol is chemically related to the local analgesics and has strong membrane-stabilizing actions. However it is used for its β-blocking action on the heart.

6.43. **The following drugs have deleterious effects on the bone marrow:**

   A. Prolonged N_2O
   B. Phenylbutazone
   C. Phenytoin
   D. Phenobarbitone
   E. Phenacetin.

6.44. **The following drugs cause hyperglycaemia:**

   A. Growth hormone
   B. Diguanides
   C. Adrenaline
   D. Glucagon
   E. Thyroid stimulating hormone.

6.45. **Conduction in post-ganglionic nerve fibres is reduced by:**

   A. Suxamethonium
   B. Hexamethonium
   C. Guanethidine
   D. Morphine
   E. Tacrine.

Answers overleaf

6.43. A, B.

Prolonged nitrous oxide administration (over 24 hours) can depress the bone marrow. Aplastic anaemia, agranulocytosis, thrombocytopenia and leukopenia are rare complications of phenylbutazone and contraindications to its further use in that patient.

Megaloblastic anaemia has been reported with phenytoin and is treated with folate and vitamin B_{12}. More serious toxic effects are vestibular and cerebellar disturbances. Phenacetin may cause an anaemia, but this is associated with a reticulocytosis and shortened red blood cell life.

6.44. A, C, D, E.

Glucagon stimulates glycogenolysis. Adrenaline does too (via glucagon) and causes gluconeogenesis. The diguanides (phenformin and metformin) stimulate insulin production to lower blood sugar. Growth hormone and thyroid stimulating hormone contribute to the diabetogenic effect of an anterior pituitary tumour. Acromegalics tend to have diabetes mellitus.

6.45. B, C.

Suxamethonium acts at the neuromuscular junction. Hexamethonium is a ganglionic-blocking agent. Guanethidine in clinical doses acts on the adrenergic nerve terminal; however larger doses have marked membrane-stabilizing action. The effects of morphine are all central — it has no membrane-stabilizing action. Tacrine hydrochloride is a central stimulant with strong anticholinesterase activity.

6.46. The following drugs cross the placenta:

    A. Gallamine
    B. Pethidine
    C. Methohexitone
    D. Di-ethyl ether
    E. Paraldehyde.

6.47. Which of the following doses of papaveratum injection B.P.C. contains roughly the same quantity of anhydrous morphine as 10 mg of morphine sulphate injection B.P.?

    A. 20 mg
    B. 17.6 mg
    C. 15 mg
    D. 13.4 mg
    E. 10 mg

6.48. What is the lowest specific gravity of normal blood?

    A. 1.010
    B. 1.020
    C. 1.030
    D. 1.040
    E. 1.050.

Answers overleaf

6.46. A, B, C, D, E.

All drugs cross the placental barrier to a greater or lesser extent. There is less rapid transfer when placental function is impaired.

Gallamine does cross in significant amounts in doses used clinically; tubocurarine seems to cross less readily. The other drugs mentioned all cross the placental barrier and will produce foetal depression in clinical practice.

6.47. C.

20 mg of papaveratum contains 10 mg of anhydrous morphine sulphate but this is equivalent to 13.4 mg of the hydrated salt employed in the morphine sulphate injection. Thus 10 mg of hydrated salt is equivalent to:

$$10 \times 20/13.4 = 15 \text{ mg.}$$

6.48. E.

Blood normally has a specific gravity above 1.050. Because red cells are heavy (sp. gr. 1.100) specific gravity is used as the basis for a simple, rapid test to screen blood donors for anaemia; a drop of anaemic blood fails to sink in copper sulphate solution of known specific gravity.

Normal values: Men   1.055—1.062,
Women   1.050—1.056.

7. PHYSICS

7.1. With regard to explosions in the operating theatre:

    A. A relative humidity of 70% prevents build-up of static electricity

    B. Rubber anti-static boots have a resistance of 100,000 ohms

    C. Temperatures below "red-heat" can ignite explosive agents

    D. An anti-static rubber has a resistance between 50,000 ohms and 100 megohms

    E. Trichlorethylene is non-explosive in clinical situations.

7.2. Cyclopropane in the right proportions will form an explosive mixture with:

    A. Oxygen

    B. Nitrous oxide

    C. Air

    D. Ether vapour

    E. Helium.

7.3. Which of the following mixtures can be flammable:

    A. Ethyl chloride in air

    B. Ether in nitrous oxide

    C. Trichlorethylene in oxygen

    D. Hyperbaric halothane/nitrous oxide/oxygen

    E. Cyclopropane in nitrous oxide

Answers overleaf

7.1. A, B, C, D, E.

An ambient *relative* humidity of 60% is generally regarded as the lowest point above which surfaces will conduct away static charges. Normal rubber is a good insulator with a high resistance. Anti-static rubber, produced by incorporating carbon during manufacture, is a slightly conducting material, the aim being to make electrical potentials of all objects the same so preventing sparks due to static electricity. In general, resistance of articles should not be greater than 100 megohms (to allow state dissipation) and not less than 50,000 ohms (to protect against electrocution).

7.2. A, B, C.

Cyclopropane can explode at the following concentrations:

With Air	With Oxygen	With Nitrous Oxide
2.4—10.3%	2.48—60.0%	1.6—30.3%

7.3. A, B, C, D, E.

All of these mixtures can be flammable, although trichlorethylene is only so in oxygen in concentrations above the clinical range (10—65%), and halothane requires both nitrous oxide and hyperbaric conditions.

7.4. Laminar flow in a tube is directly related to:

    A. The square of the radius of the tube
    B. The viscosity
    C. The osmotic pressure
    D. The density
    E. The pressure difference.

7.5. Turbulent flow at an orifice is directly related to:

    A. The square of the radius of the orifice
    B. Viscosity
    C. Density
    D. Length
    E. Square root of the pressure difference.

Answers overleaf

7.4. E.

Laminar flow can be derived from Poiseuille's equation, i.e.

$$\text{FLOW} \ \alpha \ \frac{\Delta P \pi r^4}{8 \eta L}$$

ΔP = pressure difference
r = radius of tube
η = viscosity
L = length

Note the word "directly" has a mathematical meaning (opposite of "inversely"), therefore (B) is wrong. Laminar flow is independent of osmotic pressure and density (cf. turbulent flow). However, for flow to occur at all in capillaries, osmotic pressure due to colloids is essential; this function of albumin was clearly appreciated by Magendie (*Lancet*, 1838, p. 777) and he describes the difficulty of forcing pure water through capillaries.

7.5. A, C.

Turbulent flow depends on the cross sectional area of the orifice and the difference in pressures on either side of the orifice (not the square root). Because the fluid is being accelerated and decelerated, the density is important in turbulent flow (cf. laminar flow — viscosity is important).

7.6. The pressure of gas in a bubble is:

    A. Proportional to the radius squared
    B. Proportional to the radius
    C. Unaffected by change in radius
    D. Inversely proportional to the radius
    E. Inversely proportional to the radius squared.

The questions below refer to ideal gases under standard
   conditions:

7.7.   Relates the partial pressure of gases in a physical mixture to
       their concentrations
7.8.   Relates the rate of diffusion to the square root of the mole-
       cular weights
7.9.   Relates the volume of a gas to the pressure of a gas
7.10 Relates the number of molecules to the volume
7.11. Relates the volume to the temperature.

From the following alternatives select the best choice for each of
   the questions:

    A. Avogadro's hypothesis
    B. Graham's law
    C. Charles' law
    D. Dalton's law
    E. Henry's law.

Answers overleaf

7.6. D.

The pressure in a bubble depends upon the force due to surface tension (T) and this *force is* proportional to the radius (r). However the force is exerted over the area of cross section of the bubble and the area is proportional to the square of the radius (πr^2). The net effect is that as a bubble grows in size, the increase in force is more than offset by the greater increase in cross section area and the pressure falls. For a bubble immersed in liquid the pressure (p) due to surface tension may be derived by considering the forces in a bisected bubble.

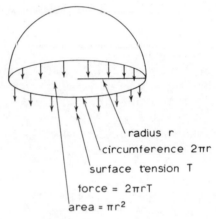

radius r
circumference $2\pi r$
surface tension T
force = $2\pi r T$
area = πr^2

pressure = force/area

$\qquad = 2\pi r T / \pi r^2$

$\qquad = 2T/r$

7.7. D — Dalton's law
7.8. B — Graham's law
7.9. None — Boyle's law
7.10. A — Avogadro's hypothesis
7.11. C — Charles' law.

Henry's law relates the volume of gas going into solution to its partial pressure.

7.12. At body temperature the saturated vapour pressure of
      water is:

    A. 4.7 Torr
    B. 6.3 H_2O
    C. 40 mmHg
    D. 47 Torr
    E. 63 cmH_2O.

7.13. Where N stands for Newton, sec for seconds and M for
      metres, viscosity can be expressed in:

    A. $N\,M^{-1}$ sec
    B. $N^{-1}\,M^{-1}$ sec
    C. $N\,M^{-1}\,sec^{-1}$
    D. $N\,M^{-2}$ sec
    E. $N\,M\,sec^{-1}$.

7.14. Atmospheric pressure expressed in cmH_2O is approxi-
      mately:

    A. 10,000
    B. 7,000
    C. 1,000
    D.   700
    E.   100.

Answers overleaf

7.12. D, E.

The saturated vapour pressure of water at $37°C$ is 47 mmHg = 47 Torr (the *Torri*celi vacuum supports a mercury column 760 mm high) and 47 mmHg = $\dfrac{47 \times 13.6}{10}$ = 63 cmH$_2$O.

7.13. D.

In Poiseuille's equation $\dot{Q} = \dfrac{\Delta P \pi r^4}{8 \eta L}$, the units can correctly be replaced by their dimensions and the constants omitted:

$$\frac{M^3}{sec} = \frac{N\ M^{-2}\ M^4}{M}$$

Cancellation and rearrangement yield the units for viscosity:

η = N M^{-2} sec (Newton seconds per square metre).

($\dot{Q}$ = flow, ΔP = pressure difference, r = radius, η = viscosity, L = length, N = Newton, M = metre, sec = second.)

7.14. C.

Considering that anaesthetists express so many readings in cmH$_2$O it is surprising that the value for atmospheric pressure is frequently not known. The answer can be calculated by knowing that the density of mercury is 13.6 and thus 760 mmHg will support a water column:

$$\frac{760 \times 13.6}{10} = 1034\ cmH_2O$$

7.15. In a perfect gas, pressure (P), volume (V) and temperature (T) are related so that:

    A. VT/P is constant
    B. PT/V is constant
    C. VP/T is constant
    D. PTV is constant
    E. None of the above is true.

7.16. The following statements are correct:

    A. The molecular weight of helium is 4
    B. Ethylene is lighter than air
    C. Halothane is insoluble in red rubber
    D. Repeated autoclaving of anti-static rubber enhances its anti-static properties
    E. The half-life of I^{131} is 8 days.

Answers overleaf

7.15. C.

Combination of Boyle's law: PV = constant and Charles' law: $\frac{V}{T}$ = constant, produces VP/T = constant. The ideal gas equation expresses this: $VP = rT$ where r is the universal gas constant. In SI units the gas constant can be calculated by inserting the values corresponding to a gram molecular weight (mole) occupying 22.4 litres (0.0224 m^3) at a pressure of one atmosphere (101,400 N/m^2) at freezing point (273°K): .

   0.0224 x 101,400 = 273r,
   thus r = 8.314 Nm K^{-1} mol^{-1}
         (or 8314 Nm K^{-1} kmol^{-1}).

7.16. A, B, D, E.

Helium exists as a mon-atomic molecule so that its atomic and molecular weights are identical (4). Ethylene is the only anaesthetic gas which is less dense than air. Rubber in anaesthetic systems which has been recently exposed to halothane will yield appreciable amounts of the drug during subsequent use. This fact should be remembered when considering re-exposure of patients to halothane. Repeated autoclaving restores the electrical *conductance* of anti-static rubber but will impair its mechanical quality.

7.17. Which of the following anaesthetic agents have a blood/gas
partition coefficient greater than 1.0:

    A. Trichlorethylene
    B. Methoxyflurane
    C. Halothane
    D. Nitrous oxide
    E. Ethyl ether.

7.18. Which of the following characteristics of inhalational
agents are true:

    A. Nitrous oxide has a critical temperature of $36.5°C$
    B. Carbon dioxide and nitrous oxide have equal densities
    C. 25% cyclopropane and 75% oxygen is explosive
    D. Cyclopropane is more soluble in blood than di-ethyl ether
    E. The oil/water solubility coefficient for halothane is
        about 100 times that for di-ethyl ether.

Answers overleaf

7.17. A, B, C, E.

The blood/gas coefficients are:

Trichlorethylene	9.0
Methoxyflurane	13.0
Halothane	2.5
Nitrous oxide	0.47
Ether	15.0

The relatively low solubility of nitrous oxide accounts for the rapidity of induction and recovery, because the alveolar partial pressure of this gas (and therefore its arterial tension) tends to be similar to the inspired tension, although allowance must be made for the carbon dioxide and water vapour pressures in the alveolar gas space.

7.18. A, B, C, E.

The critical temperature is the temperature above which a gas cannot be liquified by pressure. Nitrous oxide cylinders will therefore explode if heated. The molecular weight (44) of N_2O and CO_2 is the same. Many properties depend on molecular weights, e.g. density, rate of diffusion, turbulent flow and discrimination by mass spectrometry. Between 2.5% and 50% cyclopropane is explosive in a mixture with oxygen alone. However, cyclopropane 50%, oxygen 25% and nitrogen 25% is safe and has been suggested for use in dentistry. The blood/gas partition coefficient for cyclopropane is 0.46 and for ether 15.0. This accounts for the speed with which anaesthetic levels can be attained with cyclopropane. The oil/water solubility coefficient for halothane is 330; ether is 3.2. During recovery, therefore, blood ether levels tend to remain much higher than in comparable circumstances for halothane.

7.19. External D.C. defibrillation may require:

    A. 15—30 joules
    B. 100—400 joules
    C. 100—400 watts
    D. 300—750 volts
    E. 50—300 volts

7.20. When a nebulizer is used to add water to inspired air:

    A. Particles above 40 microns diameter are deposited in the bronchi, the trachea and above
    B. Particles between 10 and 20 microns diameter reach the alveoli
    C. Only 50% of particles smaller than 5 microns diameter are deposited; the rest are exhaled
    D. The water content of the air is limited to 100% relative humidity
    E. It is possible to increase a patient's hydration.

7.21. Medical gases as supplied have the following characteristics:

    A. Oxygen at 130 p.s.i.
    B. N_2O at 750 p.s.i.
    C. CO_2 at 50 atmospheres
    D. Nitrous oxide contains 1% pure water vapour
    E. N_2O stored at $-8°C$ is dangerous.

7.22. The saturated vapour pressure of halothane at room temperature is about:

    A. 24 mmHg
    B. 42 mmHg
    C. 124 mmHg
    D. 240 mmHg
    E. 420 mmHg.

Answers overleaf

7.19. B.

The correct unit for energy stored in a capacitor is the joule. 100—400 joules are required for external defibrillation. 15—30 joules are required for internal defibrillation. Watts are units of power. Volts are units of electrical potential. 1 joule = 1 Newton (100,000 dynes) x 1 metre, or 10^7 erg. 1 Watt = 1 joule per second.

7.20. A, E.

Particles larger than 40 microns diameter are deposited in the larger airways. Particles between 0.5 and 3.0 microns reach the alveolar ducts. 50% of particles smaller than about 1.0 microns tend to be re-exhaled. Air saturated with water vapour at body temperature contains about 43.5 g/m^3 (or 43.5 mg/l), but a nebulizer produces an aerosol (mist) which can contain far more, and therefore a patient can gain water by this route.

7.21. B, C.

Oxygen is stored at approximately 130 atmospheres (2,000 p.s.i.). In the past nitrous oxide did contain water and the reducing valve tended to block with ice crystals. Nitrous oxide can safely be stored at low temperatures: it is Entonox which tends to separate at $-7°$ C.

7.22. D.

At $20°$ C the saturated vapour pressure of halothane is 241 mmHg. This is equivalent to about one-third of an atmosphere, which is useful when working out the amount of halothane emerging from vaporizers which deliver saturated vapour such as a copper kettle or the "Halox".

7.23. In a normal population:

    A. There are equal numbers on either side of the average
    B. Variance is always less than one
    C. Another population will have similar characteristics
    D. Two standard deviations will exclude 20%
    E. The mode is the most frequent reading.

Answers overleaf

7.23. E.

The group with the largest number of observations is called the mode, i.e. the most frequent observation. The median is the mid figure, i.e. equal number of observations on either side of it. The mean is the average of the observation, i.e. $\frac{\Sigma x}{n}$. Variance is the sum of the differences from the mean divided by the number of observations, i.e. $V = \Sigma (\bar{x} - x)^2$. The standard deviation is the square root of the variance. When calculating variance and standard deviation for small groups, better approximations are obtained by dividing by $(n - 1)$ rather than by n. Each population has its own characteristics. This makes it possible to test whether one population could be drawn from another. Two standard deviations exclude 5%.

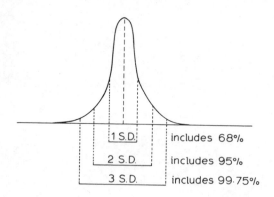

1 S.D. includes 68%
2 S.D. includes 95%
3 S.D. includes 99.75%

7.24. Oxygen in an anaesthetic mixture

7.25. CO_2 in exhaled air

7.26. CO_2 in an anaesthetic mixture

7.27. Halothane with oxygen and nitrous oxide.

For each of the above mixtures select the applicable methods of gas analysis from:

    A. Paramagnetic analyzer
    B. Infra-red absorption
    C. Ultra-violet absorption
    D. Mass spectrometry
    E. Gas chromatography.

7.28. In an azeotropic mixture:

    A. The mixture has a constant boiling point between those of the two liquids
    B. The mixture can be separated by gas chromatography
    C. The mixture can be separated by fractional distillation
    D. The halothane-ether azeotrope is not explosive in clinical use
    E. The constituents form a chemical combination.

7.29. Strain gauges are used to measure:

    A. Intravascular pressure
    B. Force of contraction
    C. Venous blood pressure
    D. Carbon dioxide tension
    E. pH.

Answers overleaf

7.24-A, D, E; 7.25-B, D, E; 7.26-E; 7.27-B, C, D, E.

The only gas in anaesthetic use with significant paramagnetic properties is oxygen. The molecular weights of gases used in anaesthesia differ with the exception of nitrous oxide and carbon dioxide; the mass spectrometer cannot therefore determine the concentration of the two gases without making a correction based on the presence of higher oxides of nitrogen formed by the breakdown of nitrous oxide. Neither O_2 nor N_2 absorb infra-red radiation as the molecules contain two similar atoms. CO_2, N_2O and anaesthetic gases all contain dissimilar atoms and are identifiable by infra-red absorption in oxygen or air mixtures but their absorption wave bands tend to overlap when measured together. In theory *all* gases could be measured by gas chromatography provided a suitable stationary solvent phase could be found. Halothane exhibits considerable absorption within the upper ranges of ultraviolet wave lengths and can be analyzed by spectrophotometers employing suitable ultra-violet light sources.

7.28. B, D.

When a mixture of volatile liquids has a constant boiling point it is an azeotropic mixture with a boiling point higher than that of either constituent. The mixture cannot be separated by fractional distillation but can be by gas chromatography. The constituents do not form a chemical combination and need not be explosive. The ether/halothane azeotrope contains 68% halothane; boils at 51.5°C (halothane at 50.2°C), and is not flammable below 7.25% even in oxygen.

7.29. A, B, C.

A strain gauge measures displacement; when a wire is stretched or compressed its electrical resistance changes and this change is detected by including the wire in a Wheatstone bridge.

7.30. Entonox:

    A. Used at 10 litres per minute may cool and separate in the cylinder

    B. Is supplied in cylinders filled to a pressure of 750 lb/in^2

    C. Consists of oxygen dissolved in liquid nitrous oxide

    D. Is stored in blue cylinders with black and white shoulders

    E. Demonstrates the Poynting effect.

7.31. In a normal gravitational field, which one of the following might exert a force of one Newton:

    A. A bee

    B. An apple

    C. A bottle of wine

    D. A newborn baby

    E. A man.

7.32. The Standard International unit of pressure (the Pascal) is approximately:

    A. 100 cmH$_2$O

    B. 10 cmH$_2$O

    C. 1 cmH$_2$O

    D. 0.1 cmH$_2$O

    E. 0.01 cmH$_2$O

Answers overleaf

7.30. E.

"Entonox" cylinders are blue with white shoulders and are filled to 2,000 lb/in^2 with a 50% oxygen and nitrous oxide mixture in the gas phase at room temperature. The presence of the oxygen enables the nitrous oxide to remain gaseous at its partial pressure of 1,000 lb/in^2, i.e. about one-third above the pressure at which it normally liquifies — 750 lb/in^2 (Poynting effect). As all the contents are in the gas phase during use, there is no significant cylinder cooling. At $-7°$C the contents separate but can be remixed by warming to room temperature and inverting three times.

7.31. B.

The force required to give 1 kilogram an acceleration of 1 metre/sec^2 is by definition one Newton. As a free falling kilogram accelerates not by 1 metre/sec^2 but by 9.81 metre/sec^2 (=32 ft/sec/sec), it follows that its "weight" must be 9.81 Newtons, i.e. 1 Newton is about 102 g wt. (or a little over 3½ oz wt.). Note the distinction between units of mass (kilogram, g oz) and units of force (kilogram wt., g wt., oz wt.). The Newton is the SI equivalent of the c.g.s. unit the dyne; 1 Newton = 100,000 dynes, a product of the metre being one hundred centimetres and the kilogram being one thousand grams. The author of this question had to be reminded that the gravitational evidence which stimulated Newton was, appropriately, an apple.

7.32. E.

The Pascal (one Newton/metre^2) is achieved when 102 g wt. (one Newton) is applied over 10,000 cm^2 (one metre^2). When 102 g of water is spread over this area the height of the resulting layer is approximately 0.01 cmH$_2$O.

7.33. The pressure in a half-filled nitrous oxide cylinder depends on:

    A. The number of gram equivalents of nitrous oxide present
    B. The temperature of the contents
    C. The saturated vapour pressure of nitrous oxide
    D. The molecular weight of nitrous oxide
    E. The percentage of liquid nitrous oxide present.

7.34. The following may be used in the measurement of pH:

    A. The platinum electrode
    B. The hydrogen ion electrode
    C. The mercury half cell.
    D. The calomel half cell
    E. The fuel cell.

Answers overleaf

7.33. B, C.

In a half full cylinder most of the nitrous oxide is in the liquid phase. Consequently the pressure of the gas depends on the saturated vapour pressure and on the temperature of the liquid.

7.34. B, C, D.

The platinum electrode is the cathode used in the polarographic system for measuring PO_2 ; oxygen molecules reaching the electrode are reduced thus proportionately increasing electrode current. (The anode of the polarographic cell is silver/silver chloride.) Fuel cells may be used to analyse oxygen in gas mixtures. The hydrogen electrode is the classic standard for pH measurement but technical difficulties prevent its clinical use. The mercury or calomel half cell is used for the reference electrode with the pH sensitive glass electrode as the other half cell.

8. PULMONARY PHYSIOLOGY

8.1. In a patient who is breathing air and has bronchitis and emphysema the following values are obtained. Indicate which values are consistent both with the diagnosis and with each other:

A. P_aO_2 88 mmHg
B. P_aCO_2 68 mmHg
C. pH 7.35
D. Plasma bicarbonate 24 mEq/l
E. Base excess 8 mEq/l.

8.2. Pulmonary artery pressure is reduced by:

A. Acidaemia
B. Exercise
C. The initial effect of the Valsalva manoeuvre
D. Propranolol
E. Hypoxia.

8.3. Ventilating the subject passively at twice his alveolar minute volume will:

A. Decrease his pH
B. Lower the ionized calcium level
C. Cause a metabolic alkalosis
D. Increase the standard bicarbonate
E. Decrease the total plasma CO_2.

Answers overleaf

8.1. B, C, E.

The PCO_2 and pH indicate a respiratory acidosis with near normal pH due to metabolic compensation (alkalosis) compatible with the base excess of 8 mEq/l but not with the normal plasma bicarbonate. When breathing air the PO_2 added to the PCO_2 equals approximately, for normal lungs, about 1/5 of atmospheric pressure minus water vapour pressure, and less than this for abnormal lungs. $(760 - 47)/5 = 143$. $68 + 88$ is therefore impossibly large.

8.2. No correct answer.

Acidaemia and hypoxia both increase pulmonary artery pressure. Exercise increases flow (but not pressure). Propranolol has no effect, and the initial effect of the Valsalva is to raise pressure throughout the thorax.

8.3. B, E.

The hyperventilation will reduce the PCO_2 and the total plasma CO_2 causing a respiratory alkalosis (high pH). Compensation (metabolic acidosis) may develop and cause a fall in the standard bicarbonate. Due to the raised pH, calcium is more protein-bound and less is ionized.

8.4. In the Bohr equation to determine the dead space, which which factors are employed:

   A. Inspired PCO_2
   B. Mean expired CO_2 concentration
   C. $PaCO_2$
   D. Tidal volume
   E. Cardiac output.

8.5. Upper airway obstruction:

   A. Decreases the maximum breathing capacity
   B. Increases the functional residual capacity
   C. Decreases the FEV_1
   D. Increases the compliance of the lung
   E. May diminish air-trapping.

Answers overleaf

8.4. B, C, D.

The Bohr equation is derived by expressing the elimination of carbon dioxide from the body in two ways: (1) as the product of the ventilation and the mixed expired CO_2 concentration, and (2) as the product of the alveolar ventilation and the alveolar CO_2 concentration. These two are of course equal and they can be appropriately expressed and arranged to yield the dead space:

$$F_{ECO_2} \cdot V_E = F_{ACO_2} \cdot V_A$$
$$= F_{ACO_2} \cdot (V_E - V_D) \text{ (because } V_A = V_E - V_D)$$
$$= F_{ACO_2} \cdot V_E - F_{ACO_2} V_D$$
$$\therefore F_{ACO_2} \cdot V_D = V_E(F_{ACO_2} - F_{ECO_2})$$
$$\therefore V_D = \frac{V_E(F_{ACO_2} - F_{ECO_2})}{F_{ACO_2}}$$

8.5. A, B, C, E.

Prolonged expiration causes a reduction in the FEV_1 and tends to increase the size of the lungs which increases the functional residual capacity. The maximum breathing capacity is reduced. The maintenance of pressure in large airways tends to reduce air trapping.

8.6. The vital capacity equals the total obtained by adding:

    A. Expiratory reserve volume
    B. Functional residual capacity
    C. Inspiratory reserve volume
    D. Tidal volume
    E. Maximum breathing capacity.

8.7. Anatomical dead space is increased by:

    A. Massive pleural effusion
    B. Inspiration
    C. Atropine
    D. Halothane
    E. Raising the end-expiratory pressure.

Answers overleaf

8.6. A, C, D.

Remember that there are four volumes and four capacities.

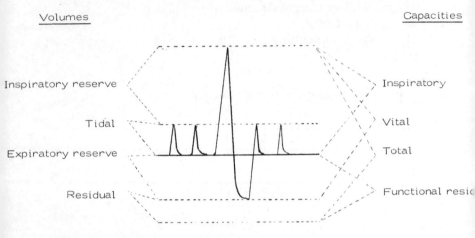

Volumes

Capacities

Inspiratory reserve — Inspiratory

Tidal — Vital

Expiratory reserve — Total

Residual — Functional resid

8.7. B, C, D, E.

A decrease in lung volume (pleural effusion) diminishes anatomical dead space (as does lying down). Deep inspiration may treble the anatomical dead space. Raising the end-expiratory pressure increases lung size and increases anatomical dead space. Atropine and halothane increase dead space (bronchodilators).

8.8. The anatomical dead space:

A. May be estimated from a nitrogen washout curve
B. May be measured using Haldane apparatus
C. May be measured using Campbell's rebreathing technique
D. Increases on exercise
E. Is smaller than the physiological dead space.

8.9. Which is correct:

A. The compliance of the lung alone is greater than the compliance of lungs and chest together
B. The dynamic compliance can only be measured during controlled ventilation
C. During controlled ventilation, tidal volume is dependent only on the dynamic compliance
D. Compliance is greater when the intrapulmonary pressure is raised
E. Compliance tends to rise during prolonged anaesthesia.

Answers overleaf

8.8. E.

A nitrogen washout curve shows how fast nitrogen is cleared over a period of time, and in emphysema demonstrates an initial rapid fall followed by a long slow fall. Haldane apparatus allows measurement of the change in volume of a gas at constant pressure. Campbell and Howell's rebreathing technique allows measurement of the $P_A CO_2$ in equilibrium with mixed venous blood. The *physiological* dead space tends to increase with exercise; it includes the anatomical dead space plus the ventilation to inadequately perfused alveoli. Anatomical dead space is measured by simultaneous recording on an X-Y recorder (during a single breath) of exhaled volume and exhaled gas concentration (e.g. of nitrogen after a breath of oxygen.) Either the Bohr equation is applied or the volume at which the concentration of nitrogen is changing from zero to alveolar is obtained from the graph.

8.9. A.

During a thoracotomy it is easy to feel that the lung alone is more compliant (yielding) than normal. The dynamic compliance is normally measured during spontaneous ventilation. On I.P.P.V. the tidal volume is largely determined by the ventilator settings. A rise in the intrapulmonary pressure stretches and expands the airways causing a fall in airway resistance but does not improve compliance. During anaesthesia secretion retention and areas of airway closure and alveolar collapse reduce the compliance.

8.10. If the compliance increases in a patient ventilated with a pressure pre-set ventilator:

A. The inspiratory flow rate rises
B. The inspiratory flow rate is unchanged
C. The minute volume is unchanged
D. The minute volume is increased
E. The tidal volume falls.

8.11. During the Valsalva manoeuvre:

A. There is an initial fall in blood pressure
B. There is an initial rise in blood pressure
C. The phase of compensation is abnormal in a shocked patient
D. The phase of compensation is abnormal in a patient with an injured cervical cord
E. The phase of compensation is abnormal in a patient on ganglion-blocking hypotensive agents.

Answers overleaf

8.10. None correct.

We are only given information about what determines the tidal volume (pressure pre-set). We are not told what determines the inspiratory flow rate (pressure generator/flow generator) nor whether the minute volume is pre-set. The proper conclusion is that the tidal volume increases. Ventilators which would illustrate the different choices are: A — Radcliffe; B, D — Bird; C — Manley; E — none.

8.11. B, C, D, E.

A sustained rise in intrathoracic pressure initially causes a brief increase in cardiac output and blood pressure followed by a fall due to a reduction in venous return to the heart. The compensatory phase depends upon an adequate blood volume and a functioning sympathetic nervous system to contract the veins, and this phase is therefore abnormal in shock, injury to the cervical cord and in patients on ganglion-blocking agents.

8.12. In a patient on intermittent positive pressure ventilation a "loop" may be plotted showing the relationship of the airway pressure to the volume:

A. The slope of the loop is related to the tidal volume
B. The slope of the loop is related to the airway resistance
C. The slope of the loop is related to the compliance
D. The width of the loop is related to flow rate during inspiration and expiration
E. The width of the loop is related to the compliance.

Answers overleaf

8.12. C, D.

The principal properties of the tracing are shown in the diagram below. The compliance is worked out by dividing the tidal volume by the pressure needed to maintain the tidal volume.

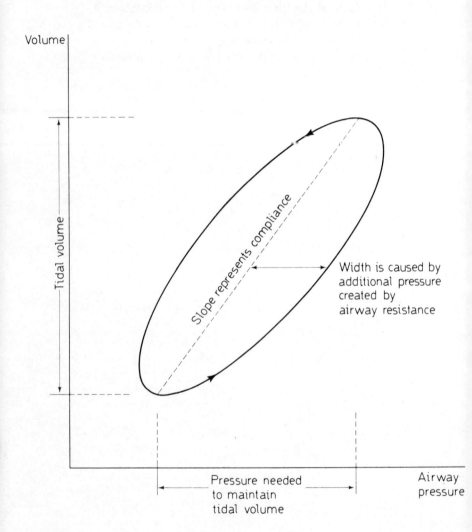

8.13. The lowest pressure to which a man breathing oxygen may be exposed without danger of the arterial PO_2 falling below normal is:

    A. 187 mmHg
    B. 152 mmHg
    C. 147 mmHg
    D. 140 mmHg
    E. 101 mmHg.

8.14. In a patient breathing spontaneously, helium is of benefit in respiratory obstruction:

    A. As the best way of improving oxygenation
    B. As CO_2 elimination is achieved more easily
    C. As its viscosity overcomes small airway obstruction (e.g. asthma)
    D. As its density overcomes large airway obstruction (e.g. laryngeal tumour)
    E. As it overcomes resistance in areas of laminar flow.

8.15. During each minute of apnoea, the arterial PCO_2 rises by approximately:

    A. 0.3 mmHg
    B. 0.9 mmHg
    C. 1.4 mmHg
    D. 3.5 mmHg
    E. 7.5 mmHg.

Answers overleaf

8.13. A.

If the arterial PO_2, PCO_2 and temperature are all normal then the alveoli will contain:

PO_2	:	100 mmHg
PCO_2	:	40 mmHg
Water vapour	:	47 mmHg
		187 mmHg

8.14. B, D.

Oxygenation is of course best achieved by giving oxygen, although ventilation will not be improved. Helium allows ventilation to rise (and hence CO_2 elimination) because its low density allows it to be more easily accelerated past obstructions and in other areas of turbulent flow. While helium's density is low, its viscosity is relatively high, and it therefore increases resistance during laminar flow. It might therefore be expected to be harmful in asthma, although the concept of pure laminar flow resistance in this condition is naive.

8.15. D.

During apnoea the PCO_2 rises by about 3.5—4.5 mmHg. Thus after ten minutes of apnoeic ("diffusion") oxygenation for a bronchoscopy, the P_aCO_2 might be about 80 mmHg. However, the action of the "cardiac ventilator" during apnoea does effect a small ventilatory exchange.

8.16. During induction of anaesthesia with 80% nitrous oxide and 20% oxygen, the arterial PO_2 will:

A. Fall initially due to diffusion hypoxia
B. Fall steadily due to respiratory depression
C. Show no change
D. Rise initially due to nitrous oxide uptake
E. Rise steadily due to the elimination of nitrogen.

Answers overleaf

8.16. D.

The "second gas effect". Due to the rapid uptake of a soluble gas (nitrous oxide), there is a relatively high oxygen concentration remaining in the alveoli. The reverse ("diffusion hypoxia") tends to occur during recovery. The degree of solubility of nitrous oxide is relative to the context of the considerations. It is fifteen times more soluble than oxygen and thirty times less soluble than di-ethyl ether in blood.

8.17. A normal adult is curarized and ventilated with a constant flow generator: what will be the approximate intra-alveolar pressure? Assume the following:

Minute volume . . . . .8 l/min.
Respiratory rate . . . . 20 per minute
Inspiratory period . . . . 1 sec.
Compliance . . . . . 0.05 l/cmH$_2$O
Airway resistance . . . . 2 cmH$_2$O/l/sec.

A. 10 cmH$_2$O
B.   8 cmH$_2$O
C.   6 cmH$_2$O
D.   4 cmH$_2$O
E.   2 cmH$_2$O

Answers overleaf

8.17. E.

The tidal volume is $8/20 = 0.4$ litres. The peak alveolar pressure is $0.4/0.05 = 8$ cmH$_2$O. The airway resistance is normal so exhalation will not be prolonged, and the diagram below is therefore a fair representation of the events.

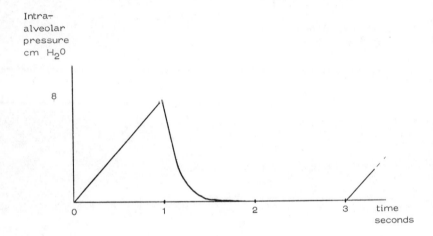

The peak pressure is 8 cmH$_2$O. The mean pressure during inspiration is 4 cmH$_2$ O. When the mean pressure during this first second is considered in relation to the overall cycle of three seconds, then the mean pressure would appear to be about 1.3 cmH$_2$O. However when allowance is made for alveolar pressure during exhalation the mean pressure during the cycle must approach 2 cmH$_2$O.

8.18. When breathing oxygen at a pressure of three atmospheres absolute:

  A. The arterial PO_2 will be 2,280 mmHg
  B. Spontaneous ventilation will cease due to wash out of CO_2
  C. The minute volume will fall to approximately ½ normal
  D. While exercising no ill effects occur in under 2½ hours
  E. The difference between alveolar and arterial PO_2 values will be increased.

8.19. An area in the lung with increased ventilation/perfusion ratio:

  A. Is an area of shunting
  B. Is an area of dead space
  C. Is responsible for a fall in arterial PO_2 without change in PCO_2
  D. Can be compensated for by giving oxygen
  E. Can be compensated for by increased ventilation.

8.20. A raised PCO_2 would be expected in:

  A. Pulmonary embolism
  B. Severe chronic bronchitis
  C. Renal failure
  D. Vomiting due to pyloric stenosis
  E. Diabetic coma.

Answers overleaf

8.18. E.

The overall pressure would be 760 x 3 = 2,280 mmHg. Although "B" is wrong, the P_aCO_2 will fall a little due to raised tissue (and respiratory centre) PCO_2. Exercise enhances oxygen toxicity and reduces the time before onset of cerebral signs to a few minutes. Some of the blood returning to the heart as usual passes through the anatomical and physiological shunts; because its PO_2 is low relative to the high alveolar PO_2, the admixture effect will profoundly influence P_aO_2. The alveolar PO_2, can be calculated by deducting the PCO_2 and water vapour pressure from the total pressure, i.e. $(760 \times 3) - 40 - 47 = 2,197$ mmHg.

8.19. B, E.

An area with an increased ventilation/perfusion has a ventilation greater than is required by the blood flow to that area. The excess ventilation is equivalent to dead space and consequently tends to cause the remainder of the lung to be relatively under-ventilated, compensation is achieved by increasing the ventilation.

8.20. B, D.

A raised PCO_2 is expected in respiratory failure (bronchitis) and as a compensation for non-respiratory, i.e. metabolic alkalosis (vomiting due to pyloric stenosis). Pulmonary embolism causes a reflex hyperventilation and a low PCO_2. Diabetic and renal acidosis are also associated with hyperventilation.

8.21. **When during exhalation in temperate climates gas passes from the alveoli to the external nares:**

    A. The gas is maintained at body temperature
    B. The gas is cooled by about 5°C
    C. The relative humidity stays constant
    D. The water content falls by about 5%
    E. The water content falls by about 20%.

Answers overleaf

8.21. B, C, E.

The nose both warms inspired air and cools expired air; it is a heat and moisture exchanger. During expiration there is approximately a 5°C fall in temperature with a 20% fall in the water content. However, the exhaled air remains near 100% relative humidity.

9. SURGERY

9.1. With unilateral mandibular fracture there is necessity for:

    A. Operative reduction and fixation within 24 hours
    B. Antibiotic therapy
    C. Extraction of loosened teeth on affected side
    D. Nasogastric feeding after splint fixation
    E. Chest radiograph.

9.2. Complications following partial gastrectomy include:

    A. Hypochromic anaemia
    B. Pernicious anaemia
    C. Peripheral neuritis
    D. Atonia of the sigmoid colon
    E. Vitamin C deficiency.

9.3. Carcinoma of the prostate is satisfactorily treated by:

    A. Total prostatectomy
    B. Combined total prostatectomy and androgen therapy
    C. Combined androgen and oestrogen therapy
    D. Oestrogen therapy alone
    E. Oestrogen therapy and orchidectomy.

Answers overleaf

9.1. B, E.

Operative interference is not urgent, whereas antibiotic therapy is, to prevent bone infection. Loosened teeth should be left to re-establish, but because of the possibility of teeth or tooth chips having been inhaled, chest radiography is mandatory. Oral feeding by straw is much preferable to nasogastric intubation.

9.2. A, B, C.

The achlorhydria results in iron malabsorption and causes hypochromic anaemia in 10% of cases. Pernicious anaemia is also a comlication because when the antrum is removed there is no secretion of intrinsic factor. Achlorhydria also causes vitamin B (but not C) deficiencies which may produce neuritis.

9.3. D, E.

Most cases are beyond help from radical excision and respond very well to oestrogens alone. Often an orchidectomy will enhance oestrogen effect and occasionally adrenalectomy and pituitary ablation are performed. Sometimes a per-urethral resection is required to overcome urinary retention.

9.4. Concerning the Bilroth I operation:

A. Vagotomy is an essential component
B. Gastric malignancy is a contra-indication
C. Gastro-jejunostomy may become necessary if "dumping" occurs.
D. It is the first of a two-stage operation
E. It is occasionally recommended for pernicious anaemia.

9.5. Severe pain in the left hypochondrium may result from:

A. Left-sided lower lobe pneumonia
B. Deep lying retrocaecal appendicitis
C. A sickling crisis
D. A gastric ulcer
E. Intussusception in the adult.

9.6. Carcinoma of the oesophagus:

A. Occurs most commonly in the lower third
B. Often presents with symptoms from cerebral metastases
C. Has a good surgical prognosis if dysphagia and weight loss are the sole symptoms
D. Frequently leads to regurgitation which accounts for the common hazard of the acid aspiration syndrome in this condition.
E. Is mainly of the squamous-celled variety.

Answers overleaf

9.4. C.

The Bilroth I is a type of partial gastrectomy. Localized malignancy is treatable by this operation, which does not include vagotomy. Although there is no blind loop involved, dumping symptoms may occur which may be relieved by gastro-jejunal anastomosis. In the Bilroth II operation the duodenum is closed and left as a blind loop with the stomach anastomosed to the jejunum; neither would be indicated for pernicious anaemia — they could, of course, produce the condition by reducing intrinsic factor secretion.

9.5. A, C, D, E.

Pneumonia frequently refers pain to the left hypochondrium, as does a splenic infarct in sickle-cell haemoglobinopathy. An acute exacerbation of a gastric ulcer can be extremely painful. Colonic intussusception in adults usually results from a tumour of the colon.

9.6. A, E.

Carcinoma of the oesophagus is usually squamous-celled and occurs mostly in the lower third. This has a high mortality and is often advanced by the time a significant dysphagia is evident, which accounts for the poor prognosis. Blood-borne metastases are exceptional. Regurgitation is oesophageal (not gastric) and alkaline.

9.7. Subdural haematoma:

    A. Results from a middle meningeal artery haemorrhage
    B. Is frequently bilateral
    C. Is far more common than extradural haemorrhage
    D. Is associated with history of minor trauma
    E. Has good prognosis from surgery provided mid-brain coning has not occurred.

9.8. During laparoscopy:

    A. Intra-abdominal pressure should not exceed 12 cmH$_2$O
    B. Nitrogen is preferable to oxygen as the distending gas owing to oxygen's rapid absorption
    C. Tubular sterilization is impractical
    D. The reverse Trendelenburg position is recommended
    E. Pneumothorax may be a complication.

9.9. When performing emergency tracheostomy:

    A. The skin incision should be horizontal rather than vertical
    B. The thyroid isthmus must be clamped and divided
    C. A Bjork flap is recommended
    D. Preoperative endotracheal intubation is time-wasting
    E. Operation through the first tracheal ring is not recommended

Answers overleaf

9.7. B, C, D, E.

Middle meningeal arterial bleeding occurs extradurally and, unlike the subdural haemorrhage, is usually unilateral and associated with skull fracture. Both types of haemorrhage may result from minor trauma and, if mid-brain coning has not developed, surgical intervention offers a good prognosis. Subdural bleeding stems from cerebral veins and the developing clinical situation is likely to be less dramatic than that following arterial trauma. These two varieties of traumatic intracranial haemorrhage may of course co-exist as may the third variety — subcortical haemorrhage.

9.8. E.

Pressures up to 30 cmH$_2$O are often required to produce sufficient visceral displacement. Both CO$_2$ and N$_2$O are used and cause less hazard than nitrogen in the event of gas embolism. A steep Trendelenburg position is generally recommended, and tubular sterilization by cautery and section is performed through the laparoscope. Pneumothorax is reported.

9.9. C, E.

In this emergency a generous vertical incision is recommended because it gives the best access, although transverse scars in the neck heal best. The thyroid isthmus is easily clamped and divided and offers good exposure. However, this structure may be ignored or retracted if necessary. A Bjork flap is a useful manoeuvre for creating and maintaining good patency of the tracheostomy track. Per-oral endotracheal intubation is normally ideal in the emergency situation because it may resolve the emergency rapidly and permit unhurried surgery. Involvement of the first tracheal ring should be avoided because of an increased liability to tracheal stenosis.

9.10. Which of the following statements are true:

    A. A cystic hygroma may be transilluminated
    B. The commonest bladder malignancy is a sarcoma
    C. A maldescended testis is often found in the perineum
    D. The appendix is usually retrocaecal
    E. The commonest bone to be fractured in the wrist is
        the scaphoid

9.11. It is true that:

    A. Urinary infection is the commonest cause of abdominal
        pain in children
    B. Acute pancreatitis is rarely fatal under the age of 40 years
    C. Breast cancer is rare in the upper outer quadrant
    D. Torsion of the spermatic cord is more likely in an unde-
        scended testicle
    E. Following thyroidectomy, pre-existing exophthalmos
        may increase.

Answers overleaf

9.10. A, C, D, E.

The cystic hygroma brilliantly transilluminates. Over 95% of
bladder cancers originate in its mucous membrane. The perineum
not uncommonly receives a maldescended (or ectopic) but not
an incompletely descended testis. The appendix has no normal
position but about 75% lie retrocaecally. The scaphoid is the
wrist bone most commonly fractured; such fractures are frequently thought to be sprained wrists and neglected.

9.11. D, E.

Abdominal pain in children has diverse origins (including urinary infection) but over 90% may be of psychogenic origin. Acute
pancreatitis has a notoriously high mortality despite treatment.
Some 60% of breast neoplasms originate in the upper outer quad-
rant. Torsion of the testis is more likely when undescended but
can occur at any level of descent. Exophthalmos is caused by fat
and oedema within the orbit which is encouraged by thyrotropic
hormone (T.S.H.). When thyroidectomy (or anti-thyroid drugs)
diminish thyroxin, excess T.S.H. is secreted.

ANSWER SHEETS

For each alternative indicate with a tick or cross whether you consider that alternative to be correct or incorrect thus:

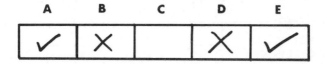

This indicates that A and E are considered correct, B and D incorrect, and that the answer for C is not known.

Those who wish to score their attempts may do so by allocating +1 for every appropriate selection and −1 for every inappropriate selection. Thus, if for the example given A and B are correct, the scores will be: +1, −1, 0, +1, −1 = 0.

ANATOMY

	A	B	C	D	E
1					
2					
3					
4					
5					
6					
7					
8					
9					
10					
11					
12					

	A	B	C	D	E
11					
12					
13					
14					
15					
16					
17					
18					
19					
20					
21					
22					
23					
24					
25					
26					

ANAESTHESIA AND EQUIPMENT

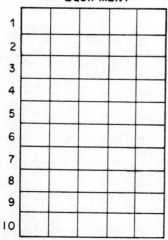

1					
2					
3					
4					
5					
6					
7					
8					
9					
10					

CLINICAL PATHOLOGY AND BIOCHEMISTRY

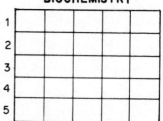

1					
2					
3					
4					
5					

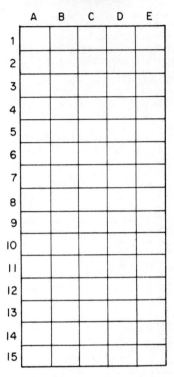

GENERAL PHYSIOLOGY

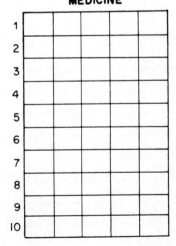

MEDICINE

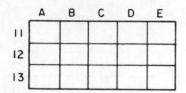

PHARMACOLOGY

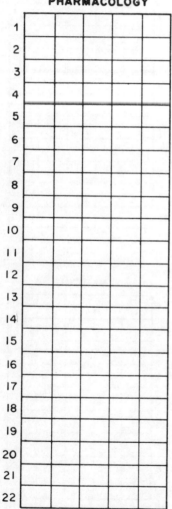

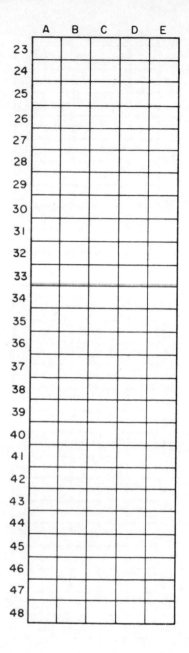

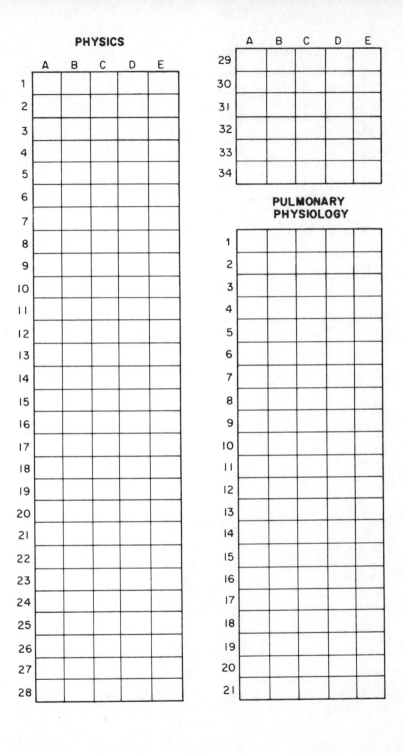

SURGERY

	A	B	C	D	E
1					
2					
3					
4					
5					
6					
7					
8					
9					
10					
11					